Sexual Health

Edited by
Kathy French
RN, Cert Ed, BSc (Hons), MPhil, PG Dip
Sexual Health Adviser,
Royal College of Nursing, London

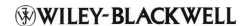

WILEY-BLACKWELL

A John Wiley & Sons, Ltd., Publication

This edition first published 2009
© 2009 Blackwell Publishing Ltd

Blackwell Publishing was acquired by John Wiley & Sons in February 2007. Blackwell's publishing programme has been merged with Wiley's global Scientific, Technical, and Medical business to form Wiley-Blackwell.

Registered office
John Wiley & Sons Ltd, The Atrium, Southern Gate, Chichester, West Sussex, PO19 8SQ, United Kingdom

Editorial offices
9600 Garsington Road, Oxford, OX4 2DQ, United Kingdom
2121 State Avenue, Ames, Iowa 50014-8300, USA

For details of our global editorial offices, for customer services and for information about how to apply for permission to reuse the copyright material in this book please see our website at www.wiley.com/wiley-blackwell.

Library of Congress Cataloging-in-Publication Data
Sexual health / edited by Kathy French.
p. ; cm. — (Essential clinical skills for nurses series)
Includes bibliographical references and index.
ISBN 978-1-4051-6831-1 (pbk. : alk. paper) 1. Gynecologic nursing. 2. Hygiene, Sexual.
I. French, Kathy. II. Series: Essential clinical skills for nurses.
[DNLM: 1. Genital Diseases, Female—nursing. 2. Nurse's Role. 3. Obstetrical Nursing—methods. 4. Reproductive Medicine—methods. 5. Sex Education—methods.
WY 156.7 S518 2009]
RG105.S49 2009   *1006475909*
618.1'0231—dc22

2008034861

A catalogue record for this book is available from the British Library.

Set in 9 on 11 pt Palatino Roman
by Macmillan Publishing Solutions, Chennai, India

Printed in Malaysia by KHL Printing Co Sdn Bhd

1   2009

Contents

Contents

List of Contributors

Margaret Bannerman – Senior Lecturer in Sexual Health and Nurse Practitioner GUM
MSc, BSc (Hons), RN Dip HE, Cert (Med) Ed
Margaret Bannerman's (previously Cunnion) role includes lead for the MSc in Sexual Health by Negotiated Learning; Margaret was Project Manager of the Sexual Health Needs Assessment of Young People in Staffordshire and is a co-author of *Improving Sexual Health Advice* (Wakely *et al.*, 2003) Radcliffe Publishing. She has been involved in a number of national projects developing competency frameworks and training initiatives, for example, the working group that developed a National Competency Framework for Sexual Health (RCN, 2004) and was a member of the DoH Sexual Health Training Group. Margaret is a part-time nurse practitioner at Queens Hospital Burton Department of Genitourinary Medicine.

Nicola Church
Nicola Church qualified as a nurse in 1992 and has pursued a career in Sexual Health Nursing and Public Health. She has worked as a Sexual Health Nurse, Sexual Health Promotion Specialist and Sexual Health Specialist Commissioner. More recently she has focused on the wider public health agenda and is currently the Public Health Lead for Lichfield District in Staffordshire. Her areas of interest include sexual health promotion and service redesign.

Kathy French
RN, Cert Ed, PG Dip, BSc (Hons), MPhil, NT, ENB 900, 985 A08
Kathy French is a part-time sexual health adviser at the Royal College of Nursing and a member of the Independent Advisory

Group (IAG) for sexual health at the Department of Health. Her background is in contraception and abortion services, and her special interest is in the sexual health needs of young people and the advancement of nurse education.

Kathy has an MPhil in Medical Law and Ethics which is very useful when working within sexual health and she is currently completing her PhD in the invisibility of young men in discourses around teenage pregnancy and sexual health. She was a member of MedFash working party on recommended standards for sexual health, recommended training standards for sexual health, competencies for sexual health nursing and is currently a part of an advisory group on the development of an introductory certificate course for primary care. Kathy was involved in South East London in the training of pharmacists in emergency contraception as the product went from POM to P status. Kathy was an author with Colin Roberts and David Evans in the drafting of the RCN distance learning skills course for nurses in sexual health.

Wendy Hallows (Nee Hallam) – Clinical Nurse Lead, Sexual Abuse South Staffordshire and Shropshire Healthcare NHS Foundation Trust.
RN (Mental Health), BSc (Hons)
Wendy Hallows qualified as a registered mental health nurse in 1996 and has worked within various areas of mental health nursing. These have included a functional assessment ward for the elderly, acute admission ward, acute day hospital, community liaison service and crisis intervention service. Wendy joined the Sexual Abuse Service, offering therapeutic intervention to adult survivors of sexual abuse/assault and their families. The service provides a specialist role within South Staffordshire and Shropshire Healthcare NHS Foundation Trust, having been developed in 1993 in response to a previously unmet need within mental health service provision. The service works from a multi-agency perspective in order to deliver holistic care for service users within the locality. The service also provides supervision, support and consultancy to both statutory and voluntary workers. In November 2004 Wendy organised and facilitated, with a colleague, a conference entitled 'Impact of Violence and Abuse' and is currently studying an MSc in Sexual Abuse Studies by Negotiated Learning

at Staffordshire University, where she is currently an honorary lecturer, assisting with the development and presentation of various courses in relation to the specialist arena of sexual abuse; a member of the Staffordshire Safeguarding Children Board Multi-Agency Training team; and a link person to EMERGE (voluntary sector service providing telephone helpline and one-to-one support for survivors of sexual abuse) which includes a responsibility for training and supervision of the volunteers and the facilitation of the monthly Staffordshire Sexual Abuse Forum.

Tony Proom
BA (Hons), RMN, Dip HE, Cert Counselling, PGC Psychosexual Therapy, ENB Advanced Award, ENB 934, 998
Tony Proom has been a sexual health adviser in large cities and smaller provincial clinics in Northern England since 1993. He is a registered mental nurse and holds the ENB advanced award/ specialist nurse practitioner in HIV and AIDS. He has held both management and clinical positions within Genitourinary Medicine and at present works as a sexual health adviser at Sheffield Teaching Hospitals NHS Trust. Tony has also been a council member of the Society of Sexual Health Advisers (SSHA), involved in promoting sexual health advising nationally. He also lectures on various courses relating to sexual health and partner notification skills.

Caroline Rowe – Senior Lecturer in Sexual Health
RGN, Post Grad Dip Gestalt Psychotherapy, Cert (Med) Ed
Caroline has worked in the sexual health field for the past 20 years gaining experience of working in the acute, community and voluntary sector. She has worked at all levels of sexual health nursing from a staff nurse in an urban GUM clinic, a sister and manager of a London GUM clinic to a HIV nurse specialist in the community. She has also worked as a sexual health adviser. Caroline previously worked as a sexual health manager for a Primary Care Trust with the key role of implementing the National Strategy for Sexual Health and HIV. She is currently employed as Senior Lecturer in Sexual Health at Staffordshire University and maintains her clinical practice by working as a sexual health adviser at a local GUM clinic.

Foreword

Nurses' role in sexual healthcare provision is extremely important, whether it be in GUM clinics, contraceptive clinics or as practice nurses in GP surgeries; the aim of this book is to provide the first stage of their knowledge into the whole area of sexual health, its consequences and its outcomes.

The individual chapters in this book provide a useful resource in raising awareness and understanding of the issues involved across the whole range of the sexual health field, it guides students into the more sensitive areas of the work they will be called upon to undertake as well as providing the latest information on new techniques and methods of working.

The Sexual Health Strategy (2001) defines sexual health as follows:

> Sexual Health is an important part of physical and mental health. Essential elements of good sexual health are equitable relationships and sexual fulfilment with access to information and services to avoid the risk of unintended pregnancy, illness or disease.

This definition shows how important it is that sexual health is seen as a key public health priority.

This can only be achieved if there is a clear understanding that sexual health does not only relate to sexually transmitted infections, as is often believed, and the clearly written and concise chapters of the book take the reader through each of the aspects involved.

Sexual health encompasses reproductive health – conception and abortion; transmissible infectious diseases – chlamydia, gonorrhoea, syphilis and HIV/AIDS; herpes and genital warts;

and female genital mutilation. Within all these elements, this valuable reference book provides information and education, the development of treatments and who are the service providers in the many health settings in which they can be involved.

Further to that the book deals with the importance of prevention and the promotion of good sexual health (condoms, HIV vaccine). Chapters discuss how to handle such delicate and sensitive issues as sexual assault and sexual abuse and the absolute crucial need for care, treatment and investigations to be conducted in privacy and with confidentiality guaranteed and the implications of the Sexual Offences Act.

The authors of the book are all extremely experienced and well known and provide a real insight into their many years of practice in the field of sexual health. Great credit must go to Kathy French for initiating this book which will be invaluable to those just starting on their careers in nursing.

Baroness Joyce Gould
Chair, Independent Advisory Group on
Sexual Health and HIV

Dedication to Service Users

In planning and writing this book, my mind was focused on the many occasions when young people attended clinics where I worked because they were seeking contraception or abortion. So many of them had no idea about what methods of contraception were available to them and some were very frightened. I do not want to recount the number of times women told me about the difficulties they experienced when they were pregnant and needed advice and help. Some women were denied access and referral to services was often delayed for them. Many of these women lacked the power and were often the most vulnerable in society. This was in the late 1970s and thankfully so much has changed since those days. Change came about because many people fought for better access, for example, the Family Planning Association now the *fpa* and those working in the service acted as advocates and raised the profile of sexual health. Sexual health is a key public health priority; good sex and relationship education matched with good sexual health services is crucial for the population to enjoy safe and healthy sexual lives.

Acknowledgements

I worked in South East London and learned so much from colleagues, medical, nursing and non-registered staff as we tried to improve the services. Much of this was at a time when sexual health was not fashionable, cool and often stigmatised. Anne-Marie Gutteridge was my inspiration.

In the late 1980s, I was given the opportunity to lead the contraception/sexual health courses at the then Nightingale Institute, part of Kings College, University of London. This was a wonderful experience and I owe a huge debt to the many students who were so interested in the field and directed me to many new avenues of enquiry. Thanks especially to Moyra Heggie for giving me that opportunity.

Over the past 5 years I have had the opportunity to work at the Royal College of Nursing as the Sexual Health Adviser (P/T) and it has been a pleasure to work with and hear from the nurses working within the four countries, hearing about their challenges, great work and efforts in sexual health even when things conspire against them. I have also had the opportunity to serve on the Independent Advisory Group (IAG) for sexual health at the Department of Health (England) and have seen at first hand the commitment of others on the group and the sexual health team at the Department of Health, always keen to listen and look at ways to improve service delivery.

A special thanks to Blackwell publishing for asking me to write this book and in particular Alex Clabburn and Natalie Meylan for the help and direction during the process.

A special thanks to Caroline, Marge, Tony and Wendy from Stafford University for their contribution to the chapters.

A special thanks to David Evans and Colin Roberts my inspirational colleagues and mentors.

Finally and most importantly I could not do consider any of the work I had chosen during my sexual health career without the support and understanding of David my husband, Samantha my daughter and Edward my son.

Introduction to the Book

This book has been written with the intention to provide an easy reference for students and those new to sexual health. The chapters are written in small bite sizes in order that the reader can read and digest a chapter at a time. Each chapter has been referenced, has additional material and useful websites for those who want to gain further information about sexual health. The authors are also acutely aware that students in some areas miss out on information and knowledge on sexual health which leaves them ill-prepared to help address the sexual health needs of their clients. Hopefully, this book will act as a source of information for those students and others who want to gain a better knowledge of the speciality.

In line with other specialities, sexual health care and treatments change in light of new research and those reading this book should check the web pages of the many relevant organisations listed throughout the book for new information. The term nurse will be used throughout the book but includes all registered nurses, midwifes and community health practitioners.

The terminology used in the book may include sexually transmitted infections (STIs) but the preferred term sexually acquired infections (SAIs) will be used except when used as part of a reference or as part of a statement by others. Client will be used where possible as those accessing services are not patients in the true sense of the word. By referring to them as patients renders them the subject to the 'expert' opinion when in fact many of them may be very up to date with their condition. The effect of the Internet has provided many service users with knowledge and information not available even 10 years ago.

It is hoped that those reading this book will think of the service user almost like a customer, often attending with researched information and expecting a professional service from staff.

In writing this book it was decided to present sexual health in a way that covers topics which nurses and others could or may encounter in their professional lives. This book does not intend to skill those reading it to be competent in providing sexual health care but aims to provide them with the knowledge to appreciate the importance of sexual health in the lives of their client group, regardless of the specialist area where they practise. After reading this book, professionals should be able to signpost those needing care/treatment to the appropriate service in a timely way and to access further information for themselves. It is also hoped that sexual health will be seen as a basic right for all individuals regardless of sexual orientation, ethnicity, colour, religion or otherwise.

It is, however, a sad fact that even today, some people suffer stigma from both members of the public and unfortunately also from some healthcare professionals if they have an SAI, teenage pregnancy, abortion or HIV. Employees are sometimes victimised if they are diagnosed with HIV and some employers may be ignorant about what to do with staff with HIV or a blood-borne infection like Hepatitis C. Employers should be aware of the guidelines around infected healthcare workers (DH, 2003).

Clients/patients who are diagnosed with HIV in some non-HIV settings may suffer from ignorance because some staff do not know how to care for them, still believing that these individuals pose a 'risk' to staff and others. Measures are then put in place to reduce the 'risk' to self and others by the wearing of 'special' gloves and gowns and often the client/patient is singled out for 'special' measures because of this proposed 'risk'. Relatives may not know of the HIV status of their relative and notice these additional 'measures', all this clearly compromising that individuals' confidentiality. Nurses and others who lack a clear understanding around HIV transmission should avail themselves of the help of their local HIV services and insist they are given the opportunity to attend lectures, otherwise patients will continue to be stigmatised by health providers who are following practices of the 1980s. The incidence of HIV is upwards and those in healthcare settings should be aware of all the guidelines available to them in order to treat all patients with respect and dignity. Having an HIV diagnosis is a major burden for any individual, but having to cope with stigma and discrimination from staff adds to that burden.

This book is laid out in chapters relevant to the speciality giving a definition of sexual health, brief mention of health promotion principles, chapters on SAIs, including HIV, abortion, contraception, cervical screening, consent and confidentiality, sexual assault, female genital mutilation, teenage pregnancy and information on training for nurses and others wanting to get into sexual health.

It is hoped that after reading each chapter, the reader will have an understanding of each topic, appreciates the importance of interventions if needed, recognise the need for referral and finally be aware of services locally. We acknowledge that sexual health training is often denied to many students, whether nursing, teachers or others, and hope that those reading this book will be enlightened enough to see sexual health as a public health as important. Poor sexual health is generally preventable and that they will be able to have the confidence to deal with sexual health questions raised that those using their services. Hopefully, they will also take time to find out what services are available locally and be able to signpost individuals to them. Sexual health services are generally able to see individuals without an appointment and would never turn someone away who has an emergency. For example, a woman needing emergency contraception can access evening clinics and in some areas those open on Saturday.

How to Use the Book

This book is presented in chapters, providing the reader with small sizes of material to digest easily over a short period of time. The book provides factual information on each topic with research papers referenced, additional resources and websites listed for further reading. It is strongly recommended that the reader views the listed web pages frequently for up-to-date information, for example, the Health Protection Agency (PHA) for latest STI and HIV figures, the Faculty of Sexual and Reproductive Healthcare (FSPRH) for information on contraception, Department of Health for policies and recommendations. Other excellent sources include the fpa, Royal College of Nursing, Brook, NANCSH, GUNA and NIVHNA; all these organisations are listed with their websites throughout the chapters and separately at the end of this book on page 217.

Although this book might appear to be focused on woman's health, this is not the intention as it is intended to highlight sexual health which affects men and women. Men are often forgotten in discussions on sexual health, this book does not aim to exclude men. Since the writing of this book the Faculty of Family Planning and Reproductive Health Care has changed name, now known as The Faculty of Sexual and Reproductive Healthcare.

Introduction to Sexual Health

1

Kathy French

Sexual health is defined by the fpa, formally the Family Planning Association as:

> the capacity and freedom to enjoy and express sexuality without the fear of exploitation, oppression, physical or emotional harm (fpa, 2005).

Sexual health is not simply the epidemiology of sexually acquired infections (SAIs) but wider, encompassing contraception, teenage pregnancy, HIV infection, gynaecology, menopause, sexual assault, male and female sexuality and reproduction. Sexual health discourses are many and we are drawn to these by either elements of the media with messages to inform us that young people are 'out of control' in terms of their sexual activity or by the publication of rates of SAIs, abortions and conception.

These messages frequently highlight the fact that when most people talk of 'sexual health', they actually refer to it when things go wrong: to sexual problems and/or illnesses (Wilson and McAndrew, 2000).

That said, it is a positive step to hear sexual health mentioned at all because anything to do with sexual health has often been a taboo, silenced or invisibilised, something not to be discussed in public. More recently and for various reasons, publications in journals have been calling for nurses and other healthcare professionals to talk to their client groups about sex. Reasons for this action include the need to reduce the high rates of SAIs, HIV infections and teenage pregnancies. It is frequently argued that the rates of infection and teenage pregnancy in the United Kingdom are much higher than that of the rest of Western Europe and action is needed to address these serious but preventable conditions. Despite these calls, it is important to note that not all nurses are equipped with the language and skills to address the sexual health needs of their client groups. Many professionals have had limited or, in some cases, no input during their training in matters of sexual health and if nurses do not have the language to help them, it is no wonder the issue never gets raised. Problems around the language of sex and how it is 'medicalised' and 'pathologised' are rife within health care. The client group may use terms such as 'down there' when the professionals may use vagina and the same applies to male anatomy with the lay population talking about 'manhood' and the professionals talking about penis or reproductive organ. Others, both clients and professionals, may adopt the language of silence and not refer to anything sexual at all. The client believing that the professional will be shocked if they ask a question relating to sexual health and the professional simply burying their head in the sand and thinking this needs to be talked about 'elsewhere', both leading to much confusion all around. Nurses and others often speak of holistic care but may not see the 'personal' issue of sexual health in this way. For example, a man in the medical ward who has had a heart attack may be very concerned about when to resume sexual activity, a valid request, after recovery or a woman who has had a hysterectomy or breast removed, all linked to how they are as sexual beings and the body image.

There has been, however, some major changes over the past few years with sexual health being discussed openly and with drivers put in place to improve sexual health for the population. For example, in July 2001 the Department of Health (DH) (England) published the first-ever sexual health strategy with the key aims to:

- Reduce the transmission of HIV and STIs (sexually transmitted infections)
- Reduce the relevance of undiagnosed HIV and STIs

- Reduce unintended pregnancy rates
- Improve health and social care for people living with HIV
- Reduce the stigma associated with HIV and STIs (DH, 2001).

The English strategy followed the Welsh Assembly Strategy that was published in 2000 and the Scottish Executive followed with theirs in 2003. A sexual health promotion strategy for Northern Ireland is expected soon. This has been delayed by the dissolved government in Northern Ireland.

High rates of SAIs continue to be reported in the United Kingdom, especially among young people, homosexual men and some ethnic minority populations (Miles, 2006). It is also estimated that some 63,500 adults are now living with HIV in the United Kingdom and this figure may be much higher as many individuals may not be aware of their status (French, 2007). The Chief Medical Officer (CMO) and the Chief Nursing Officer (CNO) asked in September 2007 for HIV tests to be more readily available, in effect to 'normalise' HIV tests with the aim to diagnose more people before they reach a much advanced phase in their condition when treatment options are less effective.

Teenage pregnancy rates have been a concern for the UK government as well as those of other countries for quiet some time and was first highlighted as a problem in the Health of the Nation document in 1992. The Teenage Pregnancy Strategy published in 1999 set key targets to halve teenage conceptions by 2010 (DH, 1999). Whilst teenage pregnancy rates are declining overall, there are areas where rates continue to rise, mainly where social deprivation and where lack of opportunity exist for young people.

The cost of poor sexual health could be reduced if young people were informed about sexuality, contraception and preventive measures to reduce the risk of SAIs and HIV. Frequently parents, policy makers and public opinion believe that if they withhold information from young people, this will deter them from becoming sexually active. It is estimated that in the United Kingdom alone the average cost of contraception for a young person under 18 years is around £18, whereas the cost of abortion and maternity services is nearly £750 for each unwanted pregnancy (DH, 2000). This figure does not take into account the emotional cost to the young woman and her family.

Sexual health has been highlighted in several helpful publications which address this public health issue, for example the Select Committee Report (SCR) (2003) commented on the poor sexual health of the nation and recognised the importance of targeted community-based initiatives, peer education programmes and outreach work. It was suggested by the SCR that Primary Care Trusts (PCTs) should ensure a range of interventions as a central part of any local HIV and sexual health prevention procedure (HCHC, 2003). Prior to that publication the Medical Foundation for AIDS and Sexual Health (MedFash), part of the British Medical Association (BMA), published standards for HIV/AIDS in 2002 and these standards offered recommended guidance for commissioners, providers and people living with HIV to help them plan, develop and audit HIV services. In 2005, MedFash also published recommended standards for the wider sexual health which outlined recommended waiting times for all areas of sexual health and these have been used to improve standards nationally. In 2007, we saw the publication of the Standards for HIV Clinical Care, a collaborate partnership between the Royal College of Physicians (RCP), British Infection Society (BIS) and British Association for Sexual Health and HIV (BASHH) and initiated by the British HIV Association (BHIVA). This document sets standards of care for HIV, regardless of the service where care is provided and provides guidance on the patient journey, record keeping, commissioning, training, networks and audit. Such is the interest in sexual health that the DH in partnership with others published *Recommended quality standards for sexual health training – striving for excellence in sexual health training* in 2005. The aim of that document was to ensure that anyone providing sexual health training adhered to those standards.

Sexual health was one of the five priority areas for improving public health in the government's public health White Paper, *Choosing Health: Making Healthy Choices Easier* (DH, 2004). Sexual health is included in Local Delivery Plans (LDPs) ensuring that it has a priority at a local level and that funding is protected. Unfortunately in some areas, funds allocated for sexual health do not always reach the intended target and the funding diverted to other areas at a time when financial budgets need to be balanced, again leaving sexual health in some areas a neglected state. Sexual health and the stigma attached to it renders it an area of health care which has been neglected over the years but the present government and those in power in Wales and Scotland have taken major steps in recognising the problem and provided funding to address the imbalance and making sexual health a public health priority. The fact remains that SAIs, including HIV infection, teenage pregnancies and abortions are on the whole preventable conditions. The provision of sexual health services and health promotion which meets the needs of the population is vital to address the issue. Sexual risk taking is often linked to the use of drugs and alcohol amongst young people and although many of them may be very knowledgeable about preventative measures, this can change under the influence of other circumstances. The Independent Advisory Group (IAG) for sexual health published a report on the impact of drugs and alcohol and recommended that any work on drugs, alcohol and sexual health should be linked together when addressing preventative measures for all three (IAG, 2007).

Baroness Joyce Gould who chairs the IAG at the DH and a wonderful advocate for sexual health states that:

> ...good sexual health matters. It is a crucial ingredient in the overall good health of the nation. If we are to see a downward trend in the level of STIs and HIV, we have to ensure that money is ring fenced; that there is targeted intervention, targeted health promotion and early testing; and that we increase awareness of the dangers of unprotected sex (Baroness Gould of Potternewton, House of Lords, December 2006).

Nurses can be a force in challenging the stigma associated with sexual health as highlighted by Evans (2004) when he stated that:

> nurses can never be immune to the influences of these sexual stigmas because they, too, are part of the culture and societies from which these stigmas emanate (Evans, 2001).

Sexual health nursing is experiencing a time of long-overdue attention and growth and this is not a minute too soon with many nurses extending their roles within the speciality. The first-ever competency standards were published by the Royal College of Nursing in collaboration with all the key nursing bodies (GUNA, NANCSH), the fpa, and in consultation with the Faculty of Sexual and Reproductive Healthcare (FSRH) and BASHH in 2003. These have been updated in 2007 and they assist nurses to progress from novice to expert, following a career trajectory (RCN, 2007). Unlike doctors, nurses do not have the same structure to help them move up the ladder in their chosen field of practice. Nurses can leave the acute sector and go into general practice and be expected to deliver on sexual health, which is totally unfair to nurses and clients. Major advances have been made by nurses in the field of sexual health, many are able to screen for SAIs, prescribe the medications needed, assess contraception needs and prescribe/supply or administer the chosen method. Other nurses specialise in abortion care, HIV or genitourinary medicine (GUM) services. There are a growing number of consultant nurses within the speciality and these leaders are taking the service forward. For example, one large service provider in Inner London (Mortimer Market, Camden PCT) has a consultant nurse as their Director of Services, something unheard of 5 years ago. Another nurse in London has set up a nurse-led hepatitis B vaccination service; this service visits gay bars and has lead to an increase in the number of those at risk getting vaccinated against hepatitis B. Other nurses have set up services in prisons, schools, clubs and anywhere where the population go to socialise. There are so many such examples of nurses leading in sexual health, not simply in London but across the United Kingdom. Sexual health nursing is a rewarding option and allowing students to experience some time in sexual health during their training would go some way in helping them for their future in nursing regardless of their chosen speciality. Sexual health nursing is also part of both the Nursing Standard and Nursing Times Annual Awards, where nurses who have developed innovative ways of delivering sexual health are recognised for their contribution and this places sexual health equally as important as other spheres of nursing but this would not have happened even 5 years ago, such is the change in sexual health nursing.

Nurse prescribing has been one of the greatest advancement for nurses and has created opportunities for nurses to be able to provide the full package of care to their clients and facilitate the running of nurse-led services. Nurses who have not undertaken the Nurse Independent Prescribing (NIP) modules can supply and administer medications using a Patient Group Direction (PGD). For definition of a PGD see Chapter 5.

In terms of preregistration programmes in sexual health, it would appear that this is a hit-and-miss experience for students at some Higher Education Institutes (HEIs); some students reporting a total lack of input on sexual health, whereas others provide excellent opportunities to study sexual health and access clinical placements for their students. This must be the way forward as students should not be allowed to be trained/educated as nurses if they do not understand and respect the religion, sexual orientation and cultural beliefs of their client group as well as the understanding as to why sexual health should be no different to other aspects of care. Sexual health is part of what is termed the 'holistic' approach and affects the lives of clients/patients, be they in an orthopaedic ward, medical ward or those having a kidney or liver transplant. If students do not get access to training, they will not be able to address the sexual health needs of their client group and this is unfair to students and patients alike. Patients expect nurses and those caring for them to be able to 'know' about sexual health or at least to be able to listen and refer them to the specialist areas. Without the training the culture of 'silence' will continue and nurses will not have the language to help those they care for in their daily lives.

REFERENCES
British HIV Association (2007), Standards for HIV clinical care. www.bhiva.org

Department of Health (1999), Teenage Pregnancy Strategy.

Department of Health (2000), Teenage Pregnancy Unit.

Department of Health (2001), National Strategy for Sexual Health and HIV.

Department of Health (DH) (2004), *Choosing Health, Making Health Choices Easier*, London: DH.

Department of Health (DH) (2005), Recommended quality standards for sexual health training – striving for excellence in sexual health training, London. Available at www.dh.gov.org

Evans, D. (2004), *Primary Health Care*. Vol 14 (8): 40–49.

fpa (2005), at www.fpa.org.uk

French, K. (2007), Sexual health: a public health issue? *British Journal of Nursing*. Vol 2 (3): 102–106.

Gould, J.(2006) Statement on sexual health by Baroness Gould in the House of Commons (see Hansard Dec 2006)

House of Commons Health Select Committee (2003), Sexual health. The Stationary Office. Available at www.publications.parliament.uk/pa/cm2000203/cmselect/cmcmhealth/69/6902

Independent Advisory Group (IAG) (DH) (2007), Sex, drugs, alcohol and young people – a review of the impact drugs and alcohol have on young people's sexual behaviour. Available at www.dh.gov.uk

Miles, K. (2006), Sexual health issues, *Primary Health Care*. 16 (1): 31–33.

Royal College of Nursing (RCN) (2007), Competencies for sexual health nursing. Available at www.rcn.org.uk

The Medical Foundation for AIDS and Sexual Health (2002), Recommended standards for NHS HIV services. Available at www.medfash.org.uk or 0207 383 6345

Wilson, H. and McAndrew, S. (2000), Sexual health foundations for practice. Balliere Tindall.

FURTHER READING

Bickford, J. (2006), Sexual history taking and genital examination, *Primary Health Care*. Vol 16 (2): 33.

Campbell, P. (2004), Nurse prescribing for contraceptive care and sexual health, *The Journal of Family Planning and Reproductive Health Care*. Vol 30 (4): 255.

Department of Health (DH) (2002), Hepatitis C infected health care workers. www.dh.gov.org.uk

Department of Health (DH) (2005), HIV infected health care workers: guidance on management of patient notification. www.dh.gov.org.uk

Evans, D. (2004), Behind the headlines: sexual health implications for nursing ethics and practice, *Primary Health Care*. Vol 14 (8): 40.

Health Protection Agency and Association of Public Health Observations (2006), Indications of Public Health in the English Regions. Sexual Health. www.apho.org.uk/www.hpa.org.uk

Miles, K. (2006), Putting STI screening on the primary care nursing agenda, *Primary Health Care*. Vol 16 (1): 31.

Miles, K. and Hammond, J. (2006), Developing community-based sexual health services for young people, *Primary Health Care*. Vol 16 (9): 33.

O'Dowd, A. (2007), Why sexual health matters, *Nursing Standard*. Vol 103 (22): 16.

Wakely, G. (2004), Clinical governance for better sexual health services, *The Journal of Family Planning and Reproductive Health Care*. Vol 30 (4): 260.

Wakely, G., Cunnion, M. and Chambers, R. (2003), *Improving Sexual Health Advice*. Oxford: Radcliffe Medical Press.

Wright, S. (2006), Partner notification for STIs in primary care, *Primary Health Care*. Vol 16 (4): 33.

Health Promotion

2

Caroline Rowe, Margaret Bannerman and Nicola Church

INTRODUCTION

To improve the sexual health of the nation, it is essential that all health and social care workers should have skills in sexual health promotion.

As stated at the beginning of this book, the National Strategy for Sexual Health and HIV (2001) (England) was the first strategy that identified the importance of sexual health promotion in the fight against increasing levels of sexually acquired infections (SAIs) in the United Kingdom. Traditionally, sexual health promotion practice among nurses focused on the prevention of disease at primary, secondary and tertiary levels (Irwin, 1997); however, the advent of HIV as a life-threatening illness has meant that the focus of sexual health promotion is now on primary prevention.

The local Primary Care Trusts (PCTs) have been responsible for co-ordinating and delivering health promotion programmes since 1999. The Department of Health (DH) (2002) published *Shifting the Balance of Power: The Next Steps*, which went on to fully devolve the responsibility to PCTs for improving health, preventing serious illness and reducing health inequalities. Health promotion activity in PCTs has largely focused on implementing the national prevention agenda as outlined in *Effective Sexual Health Promotion Toolkit* (DH, 2003).

The focus of modern public health is to encourage individuals and communities to take responsibility for their own health and adopt behaviours or lifestyles which keep them healthy. The Wanless report (2004) stated that people stay healthy when levels of public engagement with health are high, and the use of preventive and primary care services are optimised.

LEARNING OUTCOMES

This chapter will aim to provide the reader with the following:

❏ Define and explain health promotion
❏ Discuss aims and objectives of sexual health promotion
❏ Provide examples of sexual health promotion
❏ Discuss the knowledge and skills required for effective practice to demonstrate the knowledge and skills required for effective practice

DEFINITION OF HEALTH PROMOTION

> Health promotion is the process of enabling people to increase control over, and to improve their health (World Health Organization (WHO), Ottawa Charter, Geneva, 1986)

To support individuals in their adoption of health enhancing lifestyle behaviours, it is essential to have support from the wider community as well as from the social and political arena. The WHO additionally states that:

> Health promotion represents a comprehensive social and political process, it not only embraces actions directed at strengthening the skills and capabilities of individuals, but also action directed towards changing social, environmental and economic conditions so as to alleviate their impact on public and individual health. Health promotion is the process of enabling people to increase control over the determinants of health and thereby improve their health. Participation is essential to sustain health promotion action (WHO, 1998).

Strategies for sexual health promotion should be developed within the framework provided by the WHO *Ottawa Charter* (1986) which was further elaborated in the *Jakarta Declaration on Health Promotion in the 21st Century.*

The Ottawa Charter states the following essential elements for successful health promotion:

(1) Strengthening community action
(2) Developing personal skills
(3) Creating supportive environments
(4) Reorienting health services
(5) Building healthy public policy.

The aim of sexual health promotion is to 'improve the positive sexual health of the general population and to reduce inequalities in sexual health' (DH, 2003).

APPROACHES TO HEALTH PROMOTION

An approach is considered to be a description of a collection of activities, which has some common elements. Identifying the different approaches is primarily a descriptive process. Alongside this process is emerging a theoretical framework that provides a representation in the form of models (Naidoo and Wills, 1994). The approaches outlined in the following list describe the activity that is delivered by health care professionals and health promoters, who may use a combination of approaches to achieve health improvement.

Eweles and Simnett (2003) describe five approaches to health promotion. These include the following:

(1) Medical approach which aims to ensure individuals are free from medically defined disease and disability. Preventative services such as screening and immunisation programmes are examples of this approach in practice.
(2) Behaviour change approach which has a focus on the individual's attitude and to encourage the adoption of a healthier lifestyle.
(3) Educational approach which aims to provide individuals with knowledge and understanding to enable well-informed decision-making. Health education activity has traditionally been targeted at preventing specific diseases with interventions designed to prevent ill health.
(4) Client-centred approach which has a focus on working with the individual on the needs they identify as being important and relevant to them.
(5) Societal change approach which has a focus on society, taking the lead in improving our health through social and political change. It recognises the impact of socio-economic status and the environment on health. An example of this approach was the ban on smoking in public places introduced in England in 2007.

These approaches are largely underpinned by an assumption that health promotion activity is an expert led with the belief that the pathogenic description of health is the only valid one.

The medical, behaviour change and educational approaches underpin a lot of health promotion activities delivered by individual health care professionals and are driven by the need to implement national policy as exampled by the National Strategy for Sexual Health and HIV (DH, 2001).

All these approaches can be used within sexual health promotion; however, the recent guidance published by National Institute of Health and Clinical Excellence – 'One to one interventions to reduce the transmission of sexually transmitted infections (STIs) including HIV, and to reduce the rate of under 18 conceptions, especially among vulnerable and at risk groups' – focuses on the behaviour change approach (NICE, 2007).

HEALTH PROMOTION MODELS

There are many health promotion models that have been developed in recent years which aim to provide a theoretical underpinning which reflects current practice and identifies activity for future practice. Models use slightly different definitions for activity and can seem similar but also confusing. This section highlights two models used in current practice.

Stages of change model

The Prochaska and DiClemente model (1984) describes the process as a continuous one with various stages where the individual will proceed through each stage in order to make a behaviour change. This model has been used by health promoters to support patients in stopping smoking, increasing exercise and promoting health lifestyles. These are the stages the health care professional works through with the individual:

Precontemplation: The individual has not considered making a change.

Contemplation: The individual is aware of the benefits of change, and not yet ready to change.

Preparing to change: The individual perceives the benefits, outweigh the costs and the change seems possible.

Making the change: The individual requires positive decisions to do things differently.

Maintenance: The new behaviour is sustained and the individual has a healthier lifestyle.

This model allows the individual to pass through the stages in whichever they choose. It allows for relapse with the individual passing backwards or forwards through each stage.

Beattie's model (1991)

This model was developed in 1984 and further adapted in 1991. Unlike the previous model, this approach is an analytical model making clear links between the underpinning values and principles of practice. This model describes current practice along with providing a description of health promotion practice which may not as yet have been developed. Unlike the previous model, it allows theory to drive the development of health promotion interventions and is not purely a description of existing activity.

Beattie (1991) describes four paradigms for health promotion including health persuasion, legislative action, personal counselling and community development. These are generated by two axes of mode of intervention that range from authoritative (top-down) to negotiated (bottom-up). The other dimension relates to the focus of intervention ranging from the focus of the individual to groups of people.

THE BEATTIE'S MODEL OF HEALTH PROMOTION

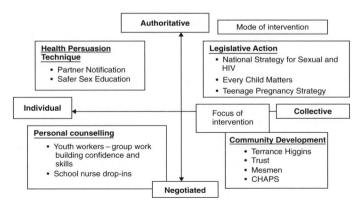

This model allows the health promoter to locate existing activity and then consider action beyond the individual level, recognising the impact of the broader social and cultural practices on health. It provides a reminder of the choice of activity that can be done to promote health. It fully recognises the approaches underlying different forms of practice as outlined earlier.

It is important for the health promoter to be mindful of the effects of professional training, beliefs, attitudes as well as the broader policy environment that regulates its content and the boundaries we all work within. Beattie's model (1991) is a framework for examining the assumptions we make when delivering health promotion.

SEXUAL HEALTH PROMOTION SKILLS FOR NURSES
Ingram-Fogel (1990) suggests that nurses working in sexual health require the following skills if they are engaging individuals to change their behaviour:

- an accurate knowledge base,
- self awareness of personal value system and self acceptance as a sexual being,
- the ability to communicate with individuals in a genuine and therapeutic manner.

These are skills that all nurses require, not just specialist sexual health nurses. If the sexual health of the nation is to improve, all health care workers need to be trained and acquire skills to ensure that sexual health provision is available to all.

The objectives of sexual health education as identified in the *Effective Sexual Health Promotion Toolkit* (2003) include the following.

Awareness raising. This can be undertaken by integrating sexual health information and education into all areas of health. One of the aims of the National Strategy for Sexual Health and HIV (England) (2001) was to improve the stigma associated with HIV and SAIs. This can potentially be achieved by integrating sexual health services into generic health services, for example Primary Care, thus 'normalising the provision'.

Information and education. Nurses can play a pivotal role in the education of individuals concerning SAIs, HIV and contraception.

The following is an example of information that can be given to individuals regarding safer sex whether in a clinic setting, school, prison or outreach services.

Safer sex

Safer sex is about protecting self and partner(s) from infection as well as preventing pregnancy, mainly by use of barrier methods of contraception: condoms and dental dams. It is important to remember that infections are not only passed on during penetrative sex. As previously stated, when you get close to someone you are at risk from picking up their bugs, and if you get close genitally to someone you are at risk from picking up their genital bugs. Practising safer sex will not protect individuals 100% but will greatly reduce the risk of such transmission.

Condoms

One of the core skills of sexual health promotion is the ability to discuss the use of condoms and dental dams, and how to reduce the possible risks of transmission of infections and the failure rate of condoms, which is around 3% per year and if not used properly this figure can increase. The following are basic rules for condom use:

Ensure the following:

- The condom has the CE quality control stamp, which ensures the condom has been made to a very high standard.
- Ensure condoms are stored in a cool, dry and dark environment. Preferably a drawer which is not near any heat source such as a radiator.
- Condoms should not be kept in a wallet, purse or pocket for more than a few hours at a time as the heat from leather, plastic or the body may affect the condom and consequently put it at risk from ripping during use.
- Before using the condom, check the 'use by date' on the box or the packet.
- Check the condom for any rips and if the packet has been scrunched up or appears rippled, do not use again as this can render the condom at risk from ripping.

- Open the packet with care, ensuring the condom itself is not pulled or ripped in the process and is not snagged by any sharp objects such as nails, rings or bracelets.
- The condom is put on the penis before coming into contact with the partner's genital area.
- After ejaculation the condom should be removed carefully by holding the end of the condom at the bottom of the penis, wrapped in tissue and disposed of in a bin after use. It should not be flushed down the toilet.

These rules also apply to female condoms (Femidoms), which can take a bit longer to become an expert at using in order that the penis is completely protected.

Not everyone likes to use condoms and, in our experience, particularly young people will use many excuses not to use them such as 'Oh condoms aren't bit enough for me' or they reduce the sensitivity. Very often this reluctance to use them is related to inexperience. Encourage individuals to practice putting condoms on and off until they feel confident about using them and suggest ways in which condom use can be incorporated into foreplay by partners. Putting the condom on and the use of varied condoms such as those with different flavours, ribbed and those with added lubricants aid confidence. Acquiring the skill to use condoms in a non-sexual setting, for example during masturbation, could also be discussed. Discuss how individuals might negotiate the use of condoms with a partner beforehand. Dispel the myths by saying condoms can stretch to hold up to 16 pints of water and the use of lubricants can actually heighten sensitivity. However, it is important that they know which lubricants can be used safely with condoms. The following is a list of what is safe and considered not safe, but this is not exhaustive and if in doubt, individuals should be advised to check with the pharmacist, doctor or the condom manufacturers' websites which hold lists of what is safe and what is not.

Not safe   Any oil-based lubricants such as

Baby oil
Coconut oil/butter
Moisturising/sun creams

Massage/aromatherapy oils
Lipstick
Petroleum jelly
Cream/butter
Perfumes/deodorants
Sun cream lotions and oils

Safe to use   Any lubricant which is sold by a condom manufacturer stating it is safe to use with condoms.

K-Y jelly
Spermicidal creams or jelly

Dental dams
Dental dams are sheets of latex (latex free are also available) which can be used as a barrier during oral sex of the anogenital area. It is also advisable to mark one side in some way so that in the event it becomes displaced, it can be replaced on the original side. If in doubt use a fresh dam.

The accessibility of condoms is very important. They can be bought from chemists and vending machines in most public toilets but they can be out of the price range for many young people. Condoms can also be obtained free of charge from community contraceptive clinics, specialist sexual health services such as genitourinary medicine (GUM) clinics, or some general practice surgeries have free condoms for young people. Some schools and colleges may have young person's sexual health drop-in services where free condoms may be given out. Make sure you are aware of services available locally for you to refer young people to if your service is unable to provide free condoms. Many of the condom suppliers will provide condoms for services outside designated clinics.

Some couples lament they will have to use condoms for the rest of their days. But if both partners have had a full screen for SAIs and they are sure that they are in a monogamous relationship, they can consider other forms of contraception such as hormonal methods, intrauterine devices and sub-dermal implants as discussed in Chapter 5 and have a condom-free sex life.

Sex toys

The use of sex toys are safe if general cleanliness rules are used such as washing in hot soapy water before and after use, and these are not shared with other partners.

The role of the sexual health professional in promoting safer sex is not to be judgemental on the sexual practices of individuals but to ensure their sex lives are not putting themselves or others at risk. Mixing of bodily fluids such as urine, blood or faeces can put individuals at risk from transmitting infections. Sharing of needles and razors, and are also risk-taking activities.

The use of language is very important when discussing sexual health promotion. The cues should be taken from the individual. Use the names they are using, ensure they understand what you are telling them by getting them to repeat back to you. There are innumerable different sexual practices such as genital stimulation using the mouth, anorectal stimulation, arousal with body fluids, sado-masochism, sex with animals, use of sex toys, and piercing and drug use during sex (Pattman *et al.*, 2005). It is advisable that you become familiar with some of the language and particular practices so you know what some individuals are asking you and can advise on how they can practice them safely. Behaviour change models such as those discussed earlier in this chapter can be used to encourage individuals to take ownership of a healthy and safer sex life and thus reduce their risk-taking behaviour.

During sexual health promotion initiatives, it is useful to discuss not just SAIs but also issues relating to general health, for example smoking, drug and alcohol use, with young people.

Chemicals and irritants

Not all genital problems are caused by infections and one of the aims of a health promotion discussion with individuals is to determine if there may be another cause for their symptoms other than infection.

Exposure to chemicals; for example those who work with materials which contain carcinogenic elements such as; machine oil and other chemicals, can cause damage to the skin. other materials can contain irritants such as; plaster or mortar, which may contain lime. Chemicals used in hairdressing and manufacturing for example, can also be irritants for the skin. If individuals are not washing their hands before and after using the lavatory or removing protective gloves, they are leaving the skin on their genital area can be exposed to such chemicals over long periods of time. This can cause symptoms such as redness, irritation, itching, pain, rashes or even ulceration.

Some people may even start to treat themselves using over-the-counter creams rather than access a sexual health service. Medicinal creams or lotions should not be applied to the genital area unless prescribed to do so by a doctor or a nurse, or after consultation with a pharmacist. Creams can be a medium for germs and may also hamper obtaining an accurate diagnosis by altering the appearance of the skin. If an unpleasant odour is detected, then the use of salt-water bathing can be used in the first instance or while waiting for an appointment to be seen. Some over-the-counter wart treatments are not suitable for use on the genital area as the skin is much thinner there and as a result may damage the surrounding tissue if used inappropriately and without medical supervision (Wakely *et al.*, 2003).

Advise the non-use of perfumes and perfumed moistures/wipes in the genital area as these can also be irritating for the skin. In fact the only self-medicating treatment we would recommend in the genital area is salt-water bathing.

Salt-water bathing
Salt-water bathing can be used during wart treatment or a herpes outbreak to aid healing and prevent infection. Place a cupful of salt in a bath; men can place a tablespoon of salt in a large clean jam jar or similar receptacle and soak the penis for at least 5 minutes. It is important to rinse off the saline solution thoroughly with clean water as the skin could dry out and become cracked. The surrounding area can be dried with a towel but if there is broken skin then this area should be dried with the cool setting of a hair dryer, taking care not to burn the skin. This is not evidences based, but some service users find it helps relive the discomfort and aids healing.

Development of services and service providers
Development of service provision has the aim of increasing access to sexual health services for people in need. This can be

achieved by working with a network of services from the statutory and voluntary sector, raising the profile of sexual health.

Individuals who have concerns regarding their sexual health often want to be seen as quickly as possible to allay fears but equally this is a positive public health measure because quick detection of SAIs can reduce the ongoing transmission of the infection and appropriate information regarding contraception can reduce the rates of unwanted pregnancies. Sexual health services need to be developed focusing on local need and acceptable for the service users.

Skills and capacity-building in individuals and communities

Nurses can be involved in this through education and outreach work. Nurses in any health setting can offer advice and support around self-esteem, negotiating safer sexual practices, communication and signposting to other services.

A specific example of skills building can be seen later. Sexual health advisers working in GUM clinics are in an ideal position during a partner notification (PN) interview to work with individuals on communication skills regarding their sexuality.

PARTNER NOTIFICATION

PN also known as 'contact tracing' is an integral part of the sexual health advisers' role, whether based in hospital, clinic or community settings. PN is a specialised sexual health skill; however, this chapter will provide a basic understanding of its importance and which infections require referrals to specialised sexual health services for PN, as this is essential for anyone tasked with delivering a positive SAI result. Indeed, any health professional delivering such a result must document that they have discussed with the individual the consequences of their partner not being treated and that they have referred them for PN if they are not in a position to do so themselves. Failure to do so could leave the professional open to a neglect of their duty of care.

The public health role of the sexual health adviser covers many areas. For the purpose of this chapter, we shall be using the term patient to cover clients and service users.

Historical background

Formal contact tracing for venereal disease was commenced in the 1940s. At that time, it was the only function of sexual health advisers to trace and bring in for treatment, contacts of infections recognised as venereal disease. Today, the notification of partners covers many SAIs including HIV and hepatitis B and C.

Whilst the role of the sexual health adviser has a history as old as the NHS in the United Kingdom, the development of innovative practice has led to forging links with other services, both hospital and community based. There have been major developments in health advising especially since the release of the sexual health strategies in England, Wales and Scotland.

Health advising is specifically mentioned within the National Strategy for Sexual Health and HIV Implementation Plan for England and Wales (2002) as essential for each GUM service, with a recommendation to create a specific educational route and registration for sexual health advisers as a distinct profession.

Traditionally sexual health advisers have hailed from various vocational and academic backgrounds, the Society of Sexual Health Advisers (SSHA) represent sexual health advisers with backgrounds in public health, sociology, counselling, social work, education and nursing. The society has written *The Manual for Sexual Health Advisers* (SSHA, 2004) which gives the full spectrum of PN and the extended role of sexual health advisers in contemporary health care settings.

Purpose of PN

The purpose of notifying partners of those with an SAI is to identify and test both those who are symptomatic and those who are not. Many SAIs may have no obvious symptoms, transient or difficult to identify, may be mistaken as conditions treated by non-prescription preparations (e.g. cystitis or candidiasis). Those with symptoms may well be too fearful or embarrassed to approach services.

In order to prevent the ongoing transmission of an SAI, it is imperative that all contacts are identified, tested and treated with haste. This will, if carried out effectively, lead to a reduction in the pool of infection and reduce health-impacting disease within the population. Accompanying this is individually agreed harm minimisation strategies to prevent or reduce the prevalence of such infections. The particular SAI will define how far back the sexual health adviser will trace sexual partners of the patient.

Protecting the confidentiality of the client is of utmost importance.

Development of services and service providers – engaging service providers to develop services which meet the needs of the service users. For example Rapid HIV testing Centre.

Skills and capacity-building in individuals and communities – voluntary organisations such as Terrence Higgins Trust (www.tht.org.uk) provide advice and information to communities, thus improving the knowledge and skills in that community.

CONCLUSION

This chapter has given a definition of health promotion, explored models of health promotion and argued about the importance of skills acquisition in order to help practitioners assist their clients in behaviour change to promote better health. The importance and principles of PN was highlighted in order to reduce the burden of infection. Further examples can be found in the *Sexual Health Promotion Toolkit* (DH, 2003).

REFERENCES

BASHH (2001) (www.bashh.org)
   UK national guidelines on management of early syphilis
   National guidelines on the management of gonorrhoea in adults
   Clinical effectiveness guidelines for the management of *Chlamydia trachomatis* genital tract infection
   National guidelines for the management of nonspecific urethritis
   National guidelines for the management of *Trichomonas vaginalis*
   National guidelines on the management of genital herpes simplex
   2001 national guidelines on the management of Chancroid
   2001 national guidelines on the management of lympho granuloma venereum
BASHH (2002) (www.bashh.org)
   UK national guidelines on the management of late and latent syphilis

BASHH (2005) (www.bashh.org)
  UK national guidelines for the management of viral hepatides A, B and C

Beattie, A. (1991), Models of health promotion. In: Naidoo, J and Wills, J. (eds) *Health Promotion Foundations for Practice*. London: Balliere Tindall.

Chin-Hong, P.V. (1993), Age related prevalence of anal cancer precursors in homosexual men: the EXPLORE study, *Journal of the National Cancer Institute*. Vol 97: 896–905.

Department of Health (2001), *The National Strategy for Sexual Health and HIV*, London: Department of Health.

Department of Health (2002), *Shifting the Balance of Power: The Next Steps*, London: Department of Health.

Department of Health (2003), *Effective Sexual Health Promotion Toolkit*, London: Department of Health.

Eweles, L. and Simnett, I. (2003), *Promoting Health: A Practical Guide*, London: Bailliere Tindall.

Ingram-Fogel, C. (1990), *Sexual Health Promotion*, Philadelphia: WB Saunders.

Irwin, I. (1997), Sexual health promotion and nursing, *Journal of Advanced Nursing*. Vol 25 (1): 170–177(8).

Naidoo, J. and Wills, J. (1994), *Health Promotion Foundations for Practice*. London: Balliere Tindall.

National Institute for Health and Clinical Effectiveness (2007), Prevention of sexually transmitted infections and under 18 conceptions. www.nice.org.uk

Palefski, J. (2005), Anal intraepithelial neoplasia in the highly active antiretroviral therapy era among HIV positive men who have sex with men, *AIDS*. Vol 19 (13): 1407–1414.

Pattman, R., Snow, M., Handy, P., Nathan Sankar, K. and Elawad, B. (2005), *Oxford Handbook of Genitourinary Medicine*, HIV and AIDS Oxford: Oxford University Press.

Prochaska, J.O. and DiClemente, C. (1984), *Transtheoretical Approach: Crossing Traditional Foundations of Change*, Harnewood, IL: Don Jones/Irwin.

Society of Sexual Health Advisers (SSHA) (2004), *The Manual for Sexual Health Advisers*, London: Society of Sexual Health Advisers.

Terrence Higgins Trust (THT) at www.tht.org.uk

Wakely, G. Cunnion, M. and Chambers, R. (2003), *Improving Sexual Health Advice*, London: Radcliffe.

Wanless, D. (2004), *Securing Good Health for the Whole Population: Final Report*, London: HM Treasury.

World Health Organization (WHO) (1986), Ottawa Charter for Health Promotion. First International Conference on Health Promotion.

World Health Organization (WHO) (1998), *Health Promotion Glossary*, Geneva: World Health Organization.

Sexually Acquired Infections

3

Margaret Bannerman and Tony Proom

INTRODUCTION

This chapter will provide the reader with a basic knowledge base on the signs and symptoms of some of the more common sexually acquired infections (SAIs) such as gonorrhoea, chlamydia, herpes, human papillomavirus (HPV), *Trichomonas vaginalis*, pubic lice, scabies, syphilis and the hepatides A, B and C. It will also look at other genital conditions such as *Candida albicans*, Bacterial vaginosis (BV) and non-specific urethritis (NSU). Human immunodeficiency virus (HIV) will be dealt with separately in Chapter 4.

The reader will also understand the basic principles of specimen collection and taking a sexual health history. As stated earlier, a sexual health history is vital to access the risk and is not about 'did you have sex'? It is more about what type of sex? with whom? and when, in effect, who did what to whom? Nurses in sexual health will find this easily and, of course, they will have training and experience to ask the right questions to get the right answer. It cannot be assumed that heterosexual sex is the norm. As such what type of sex is an important question? Clients will understand why these questions are asked if the reasons are explained fully.

There is still a lot of stigma associated with acquiring an SAI as these are infections which are acquired through sexual activity. But it could be argued that colds or flu could be acquired through sexual activity. When an individual gets close to someone, you are open to picking up their germs; so why is it so difficult to understand that if we get sexually close to someone, there is a risk of picking up their genital germs? It does not make sense and as professionals, the stigma associated with these infections is sometimes the greatest barrier we have to face when trying to treat such clients. Therefore, it is essential to do all that we can to reduce the shame some clients may feel when they are faced with the risk of a diagnosis. Screening/testing for SAIs is a stressful time for those affected and the need for them to share this news with a partner(s) can be an added burden. It is important to reduce the guilt some people may have about acquiring an SAI.

LEARNING OUTCOMES
At the end of this chapter you will have:

❏ A basic knowledge base on the signs and symptoms of some of the more common SAIs
❏ An understanding of the basic principles of specimen collection
❏ Basic principles of taking a sexual health history

BACKGROUND AND EPIDEMIOLOGY OF SAIS
Infections acquired through sexual activity have been described through the centuries with a variety of different names; Clap (gonorrhoea) and the Great Pox (syphilis) are two of the definitions that have been used. Venereal disease has a linguistic route hailing from Venus, the roman goddess of love.

Numerous historical figures have been suggested to have carried syphilis such as Henry the Eighth and the Duke of Clarence; however, there is no proof of these claims. Samuel Pepys reputed urethral stricture may well have been the result of untreated gonorrhoea, as stricture is a common result of long-term untreated gonorrhoea. Others have reminded by Llewellyn-Jones that

'[.] syphilis can affect a bishop or a 'baggage' neither kings nor the rulers of the earth have been spared' (Llewellyn-Jones, 1974) cited by Evans (personal communication)

SAIs have peaked at various times within the English and Wales culture (Figure 3.1). Gonorrhoea rates have been historically used as an indicator of the nation's sexual health, as rates of other infections do seem to mirror the trends in gonorrhoea.

Various reasons have been submitted for this. Figure 3.1 illustrates changes in reported SAI rates, which may mirror some socioeconomic changes within England and Wales.

In 1938, there was a mass production of penicillin which was made available to the armed forces in the early 1940s. For the first time there was an effective cure for gonorrhoea which showed a dramatic decrease in infections. However, in 1945, the war in Europe ended and soldiers returned home with massive movement of population (historically predisposing a population to increases in transmittable diseases). The contraceptive pill became readily available in the 1960s along with free love and flower power, also the increase in use of recreational drugs and alcohol (linked with increased sexual risk taking).

HIV/Acquired Immune Deficiency Syndrome (AIDS) and Herpes Simplex Virus (HSV) were receiving increased media exposure in the early 1980s. HIV was discovered by a French scientist Robert Gallo in 1983 (Wikipedia HIV; http://www.mcld.co.uk/hiv/?q=discovery%20of%20HIV).

Following the naming of AIDS, there was a population-wide public health programme using the media, encouraging condom use or abstention from sex. This would appear to have been effective in lowering the diagnosis rates of gonorrhoea.

These diagnosis are recorded from Genitourinary clinic attendees and do not represent the number of people who access screening in community contraceptive clinics, general practice and privately.

Enhanced testing and increased awareness of sexual health encouraged individuals to have sexual health screens, whether experiencing symptoms or not. This has also led to a realisation that there are considerable pools of infection of many common SAIs in England and Wales (Figure 3.2). Greater awareness of the conditions and screening available has lead to an increased demand and this should be welcomed despite the pressure this places on services.

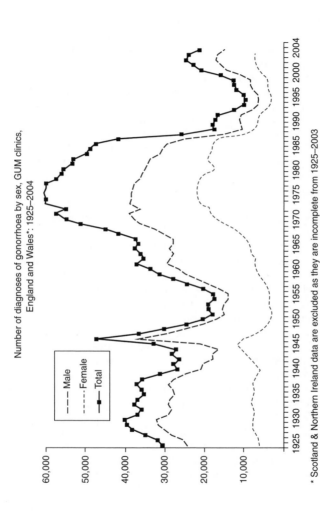

Number of diagnoses of gonorrhoea by sex, GUM clinics, England and Wales*: 1925–2004

* Scotland & Northern Ireland data are excluded as they are incomplete from 1925–2003

Figure 3.1 Recorded diagnosis of gonorrhoea in England and Wales 1925–2004. Scotland and Northern Ireland data are excluded as they are incomplete from 1925–2003. Data source: KC60 statutory returns.

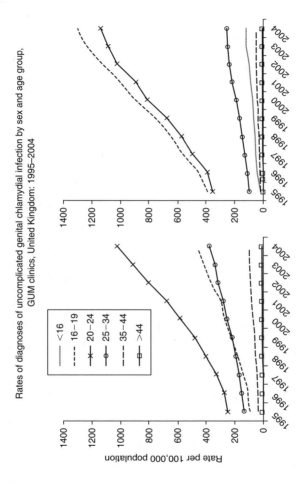

Rates of diagnoses of uncomplicated genital chlamydial infection by sex and age group, GUM clinics, United Kingdom: 1995–2004

Figure 3.2 Chlamydia rates in males and females. Data source: KC60 statutory returns and ISD(D)5 data.

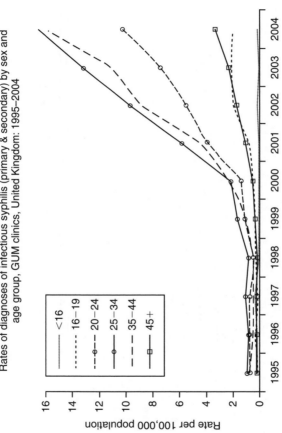

Figure 3.3 Rates of syphilis in males (England and Wales). Rates of diagnoses of infectious syphilis (primary and secondary) by sex and age group, GUM clinics, United Kingdom: 1995–2004. Data source: KC60 Statutory returns.

There has also been an increase in rarer conditions such as lymphomagranuloma venereum, a syndrome caused by a sero-type of *Chlamydia trachomatis*, and a substantial increase in diagnosis of syphilis in the past 5 years, when previously it had been perceived statistically as increasingly rare. Whilst the outbreak of syphilis (Figures 3.3 and 3.4) seemed initially to be identified within men who have sex with men (MSM), statistics show that of those diagnosed, a significant proportion of people diagnosed with syphilis defined heterosexual sex as the main route of infection, This would indicate a population-wide problem and the limitations of some targeted public health campaigns.

WHAT IS NORMAL?

Commonly in any service where an individual feels safe to ask, the question 'is this normal?' may occur. Many people who attend GUM services do so with our cultural lack of knowledge of what things should look like and as such could have avoided attending clinics. Although this is a perfect opportunity for education and safer sex messages, it is preferable that the individual is able to access this information easily.

Common presentations are men who worry about *pearly penile papules*. These are small hard white spots around the head of the penis. In circumcised men, they may be hard to see or non existent. These papules secrete oils to help the skin on the head (glans) of the penis, in order that the penis is kept in good health. Overproduction and lack of washing under the foreskin in those men who are not circumcised can lead to a strong smelling accumulation of an oily substance called *smegma*. It is good advice to tell all men to wash their penises including pulling the foreskin back and washing under at least once a day. Many men are not taught this basic cleaning routine.

Fordyce glands are another set of oil-producing glands situated under the skin of the outer lips of the vagina or the skin of the penis. They do not change or grow and are part of our normal make up. They can be quite obvious.

Sebaceous cysts are blocked small glands that can appear hard and yellow underneath the skin of the genital area. Due to the thin skin especially on the shaft of the penis and the scrotum, they can be quite obvious and as such can cause worry that they are something

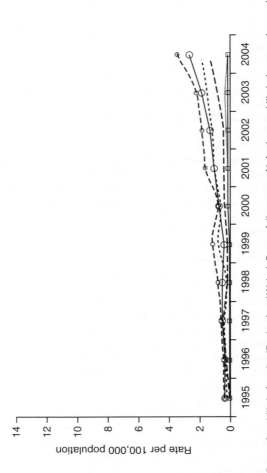

Figure 3.4 Rates of syphilis in females (England and Wales). Rates of diagnoses of infectious syphilis (primary and secondary) by sex and age group, GUM clinics, United Kingdom: 1995–2004. Data source: KC60 Statutory returns.

sinister. If they are not growing and have always been there, then leave well alone. If changing, they should be checked out.

Damage due to trauma can result in *bruising or small broken blood vessels* that give the appearance of small red spots and *lymphocele*, which is a blockage of the penile drainage system, which can give rise to what appears like a swollen vein; normally this will reduce and go back to normal as the blockage clears. For illustrations of these and other conditions see www.chestersexualhealth.co.uk.

Women, for example, may be concerned about changes in their vaginal discharge, which is common if they use an intra-uterine device (IUD) or progesterone-only contraception.

Latest statistics (including figures in this chapter) both locally and nationally can be accessed via www.hpa.org.uk (Health protection agency; HPA). This organisation collates statistical information on the GUM diagnosis of SAIs and blood-borne virus information, giving epidemiological data for each region of England and Wales.

SPECIMEN COLLECTION

Before giving an overview of the various infections, the underpinning principles of specimen collection should be understood. When faced with a multitude of swabs, it is important to be sure which swabs are licensed to obtain samples to detect particular infections. Not all swabs are suitable to provide an accurate diagnosis of every infection. Always check the instructions which come with the packaging and if in doubt check with the laboratory where the specimen is being sent and analysed for advice. Using the sexual health history, check that swabs are taken from the appropriate site. For example; if anal sex has taken place, you will need to take samples from the anus and in the case of oral sex you will need to obtain samples from the tonsillar area and/or the posterior pharynx and so on. The Public Health Laboratory Service (PHLS, 2002) (which is now known as the HPA) published guidelines on specimen collection and storage with the general rules on specimen collection (PHLS, 2002) which are as follows:

To obtain correct specimen type

Genital tract swabs
- For cervical and high vaginal sampling, use a speculum

- Avoid contamination of the swab
- For gonorrhoea, cervical os should be swabbed not high vaginal swab (HVS)
- For chlamydia, the cervical os should be swabbed unless using Nuclei Acid–Amplification Testing (NAAT) that allows a greater sensitivity and specificity, which enables patients to self swab via HVS more accurately.

Throat swabs
- Taken from tonsillar area and/or posterior pharynx avoiding the tongue and uvula.

Rectal swabs
- Should be taken with the aid of a proctoscope.

Urethral swabs
- Avoid contamination from the vulva or foreskin
- Use appropriate thin swabs
- Ensure patient has not passed urine for at least 1 hour previously
- For males if a discharge is not apparent, attempts should be made to 'milk' exudate from the penis (PHLS, 2002).

Accurate labelling is vital for the laboratory to provide precise results. For example, ensure the basic identification information such as patient's name (where appropriate), patient number, date of birth with the site sampled being recorded on the sample bottle or plate as well as on the laboratory form. Check how samples should be stored such as temperature and humidity and the minimum amount of time samples can be stored before being transported to the laboratory. Where services are part of the National Chlamydia Screening programme, additional information may be needed.

SIGNS AND SYMPTOMS
Some infections such as chlamydia have no symptoms at all. So just because a client presents as asymptomatic, do not assume they are infection free. If they feel they have been at risk of acquiring an SAI, then a sexual health history should be obtained

to decide what tests should be offered. Also, remember that if a woman presents with a suspected pregnancy then they are also at risk from acquiring an SAI and should also be counselled to decide what tests should be taken.

There are numerous signs and symptoms that clients may present with

- Discharge

Males – Any penile discharge is abnormal and needs to be investigated. It is important to establish what the man means by discharge. For example, if the discharge is only apparent during the night or on wakening, then it could be a 'wet dream' where he has ejaculated in his sleep, therefore, he can be assured that it is completely normal.

Females – All females have a discharge to some extent but each woman will know what is normal for her. However, if the discharge changes in any way; becomes strong smelling, more purulent, itching, changes texture then this needs investigating.

- Dysuria (pain on passing urine)
- Irritation/rash or redness
- Lumps or bumps
- Ulcers or sores
- Pain on or after sexual intercourse
- Intermenstrual or bleeding after sexual intercourse
- Pain in the groin, lower abdomen or the genital area.

INFECTIONS

An understanding of how SAIs are transmitted can be gained by dividing them into four main categories: bacterial, fungal, infestations and viral (Table 3.1). Bacteria and infestations are living things and, therefore, we can destroy them, mainly with the use of antibiotics. This means, after successful treatment, the symptoms will not return unless the person is reinfected. However, our bodies need a balance of good and bad bacteria to remain healthy; therefore we may not want to destroy all bacteria. *Candida albicans*, for example, is a yeast that lives on the skin, vagina, mouth and gut and is held at bay by the good bacteria. When there is an imbalance of the good and bad bacteria, it can cause an environment where the yeast can thrive, giving rise to irritating symptoms that may need treatment, so we need to create an environment where they fail to thrive. Viruses, however, are not living things in their own right. Viruses are genetic material covered with a protein coating (intracellular), which infect the cells of a biological organism and replicate themselves making the cell behave in a different way (Wikipedia Virus; http://en.wikipedia.org/wiki/virus). They cannot reproduce on their own. The only way to deal with the virus is to destroy the host cell. Therefore, our only defence against viruses is antivirals, which limit the replication of viruses. Currently, we can treat the symptoms viruses produce, such as warts or ulcers, but once the body is infected with viruses the symptoms can reappear without reinfection. It is this phenomenon of viruses, which can cause confusion with clients who can be shocked if symptoms reappear once they have been treated for symptoms, such as warts. Some people automatically think they have come into contact with an infected partner or their previous treatment was substandard.

Anyone who is responsible for the identification, management and treatment of SAIs should follow the British Association of Sexual Health and HIV (BASHH) National Clinical Effectiveness Guidelines, which are updated regularly. These guidelines give a description of the pathogen causing infection, signs and symptoms along with treatments guidelines

Table 3.1 A categorisation of the common SAIs.

Bacteria Fungal	Fungal	Infestation	Viruses
Chlamydia trachomatis	Candida albicans (Thrush) (Not an SAI)	Pubic lice (crabs)	HPV
Gonorrhoea		Scabies, Trichomonas vaginalis	Warts, HSV 1 and 2
Syphilis			Molluscum contagiosum
NSU			HAV, HBV,
BV (Anaerobic bacterial overproduction)			HCV
			HIV

(www.bashh.org). The treatment regimens and tests taken change periodically due to enhancement and development of new tests and treatments. Drug-resistant infections such as Ciprofloxacin-resistant gonorrhoea can also trigger new treatment protocols. Although this chapter will give a brief description of such information for the infections listed in Table 3.1. It is important to consult the guidelines regularly to ensure you are providing the most up-to-date advice and treatment and it is strongly recommended that you print off a hard copy of the Clinical Effectiveness Guidelines (www.bashh.org).

It has not been possible to reproduce colour photographs for this book. However, it is possible to view illustrations of the following infections and other normal and abnormal conditions at www.chestersexualhealth.co.uk.

BACTERIAL INFECTIONS

Chlamydia trachomatis
Chlamydia is the most common curable SAI. Individuals do not need to have penetrative sex as the bacteria can be transferred from one mucous site to another, such as the eyes, throat, anus, vagina, cervix or urethra. It is estimated that between 5% and 10% of sexually active females under the age of 24 and sexually active males aged between 20 and 24 years may be infected (www.hpa.org).

Signs and symptoms
Up to 70% of women and 50% of men will be asymptomatic but if symptoms do occur they can include urethral discharge and dysuria for men and post-coital or intermenstrual bleeding, lower abdominal pain, increase discharge, mucopurulent cervicitis, contact bleeding and dysuria for women. However, these symptoms may be so mild that the patient may not even notice. There may be some discomfort and discharge in anal infections but are mainly asymptomatic as are pharyngeal infections. Women using contraception may complain of intramenstrual bleeding and the possibility of chlamydia should be considered.

Diagnosis

Diagnosis in women is by taking a sample from the cervix using a speculum examination as the sample must contain cervical columnar cells and be tested using the NAAT technique, which is currently the most sensitive and specific test for *Chlamydia trachomatis*. For men, a urine sample using the first catch urine can be used when using the NAAT testing. If any other form of test is used, consult the Clinical Effectiveness Guidelines (www.bashh.org).

Treatment

Treatment is by antibiotics to destroy the bacteria. The recommendations can change as to the particular antibiotics; so it is important to check the Clinical Effectiveness Guidelines to check what the up-to-date recommendations are (www.bashh.org). Provided all partners are also treated, the infection should not reoccur unless the client is reinfected. See Partner Notification (Chapter 2; Pattman *et al.*, 2007).

Neisseria gonorrhoea

Aetiology

Gonorrhoea is an infection with the Gram negative Diplococcus bacteria *Neisseria gonorrhoea*. Again, individuals do not need to have penetrative sex as the bacteria can be transferred from one mucous site to another, such as the eyes, throat, anus, vagina, cervix or urethra. It can also invade open wounds such as cuts and grazes. Gonorrhoea is the second most common bacterial SAI in the United Kingdom with 22,335 infections diagnosed in GUM clinics in 2004. It is most common in young people, with males aged 20–24 years and females aged 16–19 years (www.hpa.org.uk).

Signs and symptoms

Not all women will present with symptoms but this is less likely in men. The most common symptoms are discharge and dysuria in men and increased vaginal discharge and dysuria in women. Rectal, endocervical and pharyngeal infections are usually asymptomatic.

Diagnosis

Diagnosis can be by sampling the infected site using a culture medium. The PHLS (2002) states that the gaining of the ideal specimen with the use of culture media for the testing of gonorrhoea are as follows:

The ideal specimen for gonorrhoea should be:

- Inoculation made directly on to culture media at the bedside and incubated without delay
- Record on transport medium origin of specimen
- Specimens transported and processed ASAP but within 48 hours (PHLS, 2002).

NAAT testing can also be used for testing the endocervix or urethra but there are currently no NAAT tests available for anal or pharyngeal sites.

Treatment

Treatment is by antibiotics, which destroy the bacteria but Gonorrhoea has a tendency to become immune against some antibiotics and culture and sensitivity may be necessary to identify which antibiotics will be sensitive to that particular infection. Consult the Clinical Effectiveness Guidelines (www.bashh.org) on what is the current recommendation for treatment. Provided all partners are also treated, the infection should not reoccur unless the client is reinfected. See Partner Notification (Chapter 2).

Pelvic inflammatory disease – not an SAI

Aetiology

Contrary to popular belief, pelvic inflammatory disease (PID) is not an SAI in its own right. It is an inflammation in the pelvic area which could incorporate the ovaries, fallopian tubes, parametrium and pelvic peritoneum. It is caused by an undiagnosed infection, which could be an SAI such as chlamydia or gonorrhoea but could also be caused by other infections such as streptococci bacteria.

Signs and symptoms

PID may be asymptomatic and only discovered under infertility investigations. However, symptoms may include:

- Lower abdominal pain or tenderness, which can be severe in an acute episode
- Abnormal bleeding
- Vaginal discharge
- Menstrual irregularity
- Dysmenorrhoea (painful periods)
- Nausea and vomiting.

Treatment

PID is an emergency condition needing appropriate investigations. Women should be seen by a gynaecologist to ensure correct diagnosis.

PID if left untreated can cause scarring and ultimately affect fertility. The management and treatment is determined by the identification of the causative bacteria. Consult the Clinical Effectiveness Guidelines (www.bashh.org) on what is the current recommendation for treatment (Pattman *et al.*, 2007).

It is occasionally reported that women with an IUD attend an Accident and Emergency department with mild abdominal pain and are diagnosed with PID. The woman is given antibiotics and the IUD removed with no other contraception advised/offered and she finds herself pregnant within a few months. It is important that an accurate diagnosis is made as not all abdominal pain is PID.

Syphilis

Aetiology

Syphilis is an infection of the spirochaete bacterium. Transmission is by direct contact of an infectious lesion, direct transmission between mother and child during pregnancy or via infected blood products. Syphilis increased sharply in the 1990s. Between 1995 and 2003, the incidents of newly diagnosed syphilis infections in GUM had increased by 1058%. However, in the following 2 years, there was a 1% drop (www.hpa.org.uk). Although still relatively low numbers, such steep rises must be cause for concern. The figures were highest in MSM. Syphilis is classified into acquired or congenital. Acquired can be described in three stages: as early, late and early latent, with early including the primary and secondary stages and early latent is within 2 years of being infected. Late is after the first 2 years of infection and includes the tertiary stage. Congenital syphilis is classified into early and late, with early being a diagnosis in the first 2 years of life and late being a diagnosis from 2 years onwards.

Signs and symptoms

The symptoms of primary syphilis is the appearance of a chancre which is an ulcer that develops at the point of infection, normally within a month of being exposed, where the spirochaetes enter the body, typically in the anogenital area when transmitted during sexual intercourse but can also be on the tongue transmitted during oral sex and even fingers. Normally a single chancre would appear, generally painless and can be discharging a clear serum. These chancres are extremely infectious and teeming with spirochaetes. The chancres will normally clear-up within a few weeks. The spirochaetes then start to move throughout the body giving rise to the symptoms of secondary syphilis, normally within the first 2 years of being infected, which is typified by a rash, normally starting on the palms and soles of the feet, spreading throughout the body. This rash is not normally itchy and is painless. Flat, warty-like growths can appear on the vulva in women and the anus in both sexes. This is normally accompanied by flu-like symptoms, loss of appetite, tiredness and swollen glands. White patches in the mouth and tongue can appear and occasionally patchy hair loss. This stage is also very infectious and can last up to several months. The infection then enters a latent period which can last many years where on the surface it would appear nothing much is happening but the individual is still infectious. If untreated, the spirochaetes start attacking the central nervous system, the heart, brain, eyes, bones and other internal organs. This is when syphilis could prove fatal. This is known as the tertiary stage.

In congenital syphilis, symptoms do not normally appear in the first 2 weeks of life. Failure to thrive, snuffly, sores in the mouth and nose. A rash, similar to that of secondary syphilis around the mouth, anogenital area, palms and soles of the feet may occur. Hair can be sparse with brittle, atrophic nails. General malaise, swollen glands and anaemia can also be present. Some orthopaedic problems may be present along with other more serious complications such as meningitis. Late congenital syphilis will be asymptomatic in the majority of cases, however, the symptoms of early syphilis may cause complications such as deafness, damage to the joints, malformations to the face often described as a bulldog appearance, the bones of the arms and legs may have nodules and may be bowed.

Diagnosis
Diagnosis is normally by serology; a blood test but swabs of the chancre may also support the serology. All pregnant women are offered screening for syphilis to reduce the chances of congenital syphilis.

Treatment
Treatment is by antibiotics, which is very effective in the primary and secondary stages providing an effective cure by killing the bacteria but this is less likely in the latent period and normally incurable by the tertiary stage. Consult the Clinical Effectiveness Guidelines (www.bashh.org) on what is the current recommendation for treatment. When cured, provided all partners are also treated the infection should not reoccur unless the patient is reinfected. See Partner Notification (Chapter 2; Pattman *et al.*, 2007)

Non-specific urethritis/cervicitis

Aetiology
Non-specific Urethritis (NSU) is an inflammation of the male urethra which can be caused by a number of different infections but typically by SAIs and is mainly described as gonococcal when *Neisseria gonorrhoea* is detected or non-gonococcal (NGU) when absent. The female equivalent of NSU is mucopurulent cervicitis. Of the NGU infections, 40% of cases reported are as a result of chlamydia infection (www.bashh.org). However, rarely

it can be a result of an allergic reaction to chemicals or bubble baths for example or a non-SAI such as cystitis.

Signs and symptoms
Can be asymptomatic

- Dysuria
- A white or cloudy penile discharge, particularly in the morning
- Penile irritation
- Increased frequency in the passing of urine.

Diagnosis
Samples are taken by a urethral swab and examined under a microscope using a Gram-stained plate to identify the presence of pus cells. A positive chlamydia or conococcal test might reveal the cause of the NSU. Urine samples can also be taken and tested for the presence of an infection.

Treatment
Treatment is based on the identification of the infection caus-ing NSU. But mainly it is by antibiotics. Consult the Clinical Effectiveness Guidelines (www.bashh.org) on what is the current recommendation for treatment. When cured, provided all part-ners are also treated the infection should not reoccur unless the patient is reinfected. See Partner Notification (Chapter 2; Pattman *et al.*, 2007).

BV – not an SAI

Aetiology
BV is an extremely common vaginal infection caused by an over-growth of anaerobic organisms in the vagina which replaces the naturally present lactobacilli and increases the pH which becomes more alkaline, from less than pH 4.5 up to pH 7.0. Men cannot get BV and is not considered an SAI. The cause is, nor-mally, when something happens to upset the natural equilibrium of the vagina that could be an increase in sexual activity, over use of scented soaps or medication such as antibiotics. Hormonal

changes during the menstrual cycle, semen after unprotected sex, smoking and those women who are fitted with an IUD and genetic factors may also play a part, as it is more common in black women than white. It may be a common practice for women from some cultures to douche with dettol that should be discussed and the woman should be advised to refrain from this practice.

Signs and symptoms
- Many women are asymptomatic.
- Symptoms are characterised by an offensive fishy-smelling discharge.

Diagnosis
Diagnosis is via an HVS which is sent to the laboratory or by a vaginal smeared Gram-stained plate being examined under the microscope.

Treatment
BV may well clear-up by itself. However, as there is a correlation between late miscarriages and pre-term births, it is vital that early detection and treatment is obtained in pregnant women. Consult the Clinical Effectiveness Guidelines (www.bashh.org) on what is the current recommendation for treatment. BV is not an SAI so there is no need for Partner Notification (Pattman *et al.*, 2007).

FUNGAL INFECTIONS

Thrush (*Vulvovaginal candidiasis*)

Aetiology
Thrush is a common infection caused by a yeast infection, most commonly by the *Candida albicans* species; a less likely cause is the non-albican species such as *Candida glabrata*, which lives harmlessly on the skin, gut, vagina and in the mouth and kept in check by harmless bacteria. However, when the balance of this bacterium is disturbed, it creates an environment where the yeast thrives giving rise to irritating symptoms.

Signs and symptoms

Signs and symptoms include the following:

- Itching/irritation
- Soreness
- Creamy, thick cottage cheese-like vaginal discharge
- Dysuria
- Pain during sexual intercourse
- Swelling
- Fissures.

Diagnosis

Swabs will be taken from the vagina and looked under a microscope on a Gram-stained plate. The identification of spores or pseudohyphae will provide a positive diagnosis.

Treatment

Consult the Clinical Effectiveness Guidelines (www.bashh.org) on what is the current recommendation for treatment (Pattman *et al.*, 2007).

INFESTATIONS

Pubic lice (crabs)

Aetiology

Pubic lice are wingless insects which cannot jump or fly and although part of the same family are different from head or body lice, being smaller and squatter. When viewed under a microscope, the pincers can be easily distinguished thereby providing pubic lice with their nickname 'crabs'. The life cycle of a pubic louse is in the followingthree stages:

- The nit – This is the oval egg in which the lice begins life and moves away from the skin as the hair grows.
- The nymph – The baby lice breaks free from the egg by releasing air from its anus and moves back to the hair root to feed on blood.

- The matured lice – This is approximately 1–2 mm in length and dark grey to brown in colour. It has three pairs of legs with claws designed to grasp the hair. Head lice claws are smaller to grasp the finer hair on the head. They feed off the blood and may feed off the same spot for days. Passed by direct skin to skin contact but it is possible to pick them up from infected bedding, clothes or towels but less likely. However, lice will not survive without their food source of blood for more than 24–48 hours. Pubic lice may also be found on eyelashes and it has also been known that pubic lice can be passed from nipple hair to babies' eyes during breast-feeding.

Signs and symptoms
- Intense irritation
- Black spots in the genital area or underwear may indicate lice faecal matter
- 'Bite marks' may be visible indicating feeding sites
- In the case of eye lash infestation conjunctivitis symptoms may occur.

Diagnosis
- Can be seen with the naked eye
- Black spots or bite marks on the skin
- Movement of the lice can be detected under the microscope.

Treatment
Treatment is by a lotion, consult the Clinical Effectiveness Guidelines (www.bashh.org) on what is the current recommendation for treatment. The lotion should be applied to the entire body. Ensure that clothes, towels and bed-linen are washed in at least 50°C. When cured, provided the partner(s) are also treated the infection should not reoccur unless the client is reinfected. See Partner Notification (Chapter 2; Pattman *et al.*, 2007).

Scabies

Aetiology
Scabies is caused by a small mite, which cannot be seen by the naked eye and burrows under the skin. It is spread from person

to person by close physical contact, including hand-holding. It is also possible, although less likely by infected bed-linen, towels and clothes.

Signs and symptoms
- Itching, particularly at night
- Rash or tiny spots between and on the sides of the fingers, wrists, armpits, abdomen, breasts, genitals and buttocks.

Diagnosis
Diagnosis is possible by visualising the characteristic rash or spots. A flake of skin can be put on a plate and examined under a microscope and a louse may be seen.

Treatment
Treatment is by a lotion, consult the Clinical Effectiveness Guidelines (www.bashh.org) on what is the current recommendation for treatment. The lotion should be applied to the entire body. Ensure that clothes, towels and bed-linen are washed in at least 50°C. When cured, provided all partners are also treated and clothes and bed-linen washed thoroughly, the infection should not reoccur unless the client is reinfected. See Partner Notification (Chapter 2; Pattman *et al.*, 2007).

Trichomonas vaginalis

Aetiology
Trichomonas vaginalis is caused by a tiny parasite and is generally passed from one person to another during sexual contact via genital excretions. In women, it is found in the vagina and urethra and in the urethra in men. It can also be passed from mother to baby during delivery. It has been known for *Trichomonas* to survive in warm, damp atmospheres such as steam rooms.

Signs and symptoms
- Can be asymptomatic
- Characterised by a frothy white vaginal discharge in women and a thin whitish discharge in men

- Dysuria
- Pain during sexual intercourse
- Lower abdominal tenderness
- Soreness and/or irritation.

Diagnosis

A swab of the vagina and the urethra in men is taken and examined under a microscope on a 'wet plate' and needs to be examined immediately. Alternatively, a generic transport medium may be used and inoculate a growth medium within 24 hours or a first catch urine may also be cultured.

Treatment

Treatment is by antibiotics. Consult the Clinical Effectiveness Guidelines (www.bashh.org) on what is the current recommendation for treatment. When cured, provided all partners are also treated the infection should not reoccur unless the patient is reinfected. See Partner Notification (Chapter 2; Pattman *et al.*, 2007).

VIRUSES

HPV warts

Aetiology

Anogenital warts are caused by the HPV. Up-to-date of over 100 different genotypes of the virus have been identified and are classified numerically. Types 18 and 16 have been detected in anogenital squamous cell carcinomas and are described as oncogenic (high risk). The remainder are described as non-oncogenic (low risk), however, types 6 and 11 are the types most likely to be the cause of anogenital warts. The virus is transferred from person to person by direct skin contact, most commonly when a lesion is present, also from genital fluids infected by the virus and may also be transmitted from mother to child during delivery.

Signs and symptoms

Small fleshy growths sometimes described as lesions appear at or near the site where the virus enters the basal layers of the epithelium. It has also been known that digital warts have been transmitted to another's genital area. They can appear cauli-flower like and found in the warm moist and hair free areas of the skin, or they can appear more keratanised in the dryer areas of the anogenital skin. Alternatively, they may appear as smooth papules, particularly on the penile shaft.

Diagnosis

Diagnosis is usually by clinical appearance. A proctoscope should be used to examine and check for anal warts, and for speculum examination to identify vaginal or cervical warts. Skin biopsy would confirm diagnosis but is not normally found to be necessary.

Treatment

As with all viruses there are no tablets or injections that can be given to destroy the virus without destroying the host cell. Treatment for viruses is limited to antivirals, which limit the replication of the virus until the immune system can suppress it enough for the symptoms to disappear. The HPV virus 'stores itself' in the infected area and when the immune system is depressed in the future via, fighting off another infection, smoking, or stress, the symptoms may reappear. Clients sometimes fear they have been reinfected or have not been treated properly on the first outbreak, when in fact a depleted immune system has allowed the symptoms to recur. Treatment is available to treat the symptoms, with the latest recommended treatments being found in the Clinical Effectiveness Guidelines (www.bashh.org; Pattman *et al.*, 2007).

HSV type 1 and type 2

Aetiology

Herpes is caused by the HSV and can affect the mouth, nose, anogenital area or fingers. The virus is categorised into two types; type 1 which normally infects the mouth or nose and type 2 which infects the genital area. However, it is possible for the anogenital area to be infected by type 1 during oral sex or vice versa. It is transmitted via skin to skin transmission particularly where there is an abrasive action or rubbing of the skin is involved such as kissing or during sexual activity. The virus requires a damp moist atmosphere to survive and will not live very long outside the body. However, it is possible for the virus to be stored in a warm damp towel and then transmitted when another uses it to rub themselves dry. Therefore, it is recommended that individuals keep to their own towels, particularly during an outbreak and then wash them in a minimum of 50°C. The virus enters the body at the site of infection and stores itself in the nerve fibres under the skin. In some cases, it will not cause any symptoms until the virus is activated by a depleted immune system.

It is possible for virus shedding to occur when the client is asymptomatic. This gets less likely as time goes on.

Signs and symptoms

An itching or tingling at the affected site is normally the first sign of an outbreak. Sometimes the immune system can fight the virus and this is the only symptom that occurs. Or alternatively if antivirals can be taken at this time, this may also hold back any further symptoms.

Small blisters then appear which are filled with a fluid which burst leaving ulcerated skin. These ulcers are normally very painful and clients report it is very painful to pass urine and often reduce fluid intake as a consequence. This is the worst possible thing they could do. They should be encouraged to increase their fluid intake to dilute their urine as much as possible. Urinating into water, a couple of inches in the bath for women or a jam jar for men will also reduce the pain of passing urine.

Eventually the ulcers dry and scab over before healing up altogether. The first outbreak is normally the most severe and can take up to 4 weeks for the ulcers to heal up. It is during this time that the virus is at its most contagious.

Flu-like symptoms are also reported as the body tries to fight the virus.

Diagnosis

Diagnosis is via a swab of the ulcerated site and transported via viral cell medium which should be kept at 4°C. There is serology available but this is of limited value as it only detects antibodies.

Treatment

Again as with the HPV virus, there are no tablets or injections that can be given to inactivate the virus without destroying the host cell. The HSV virus 'stores itself' in the nerve fibres supplying the infected area and when the immune system is depressed in the future via, fighting off another infection, smoking, or stress, the symptoms may reappear. Local nerve stimulation such as trauma or ultraviolet light can also reactivate the virus. Clients sometimes fear they have been reinfected or have not been treated properly on the first outbreak, when in fact a depleted immune system has allowed the symptoms to recur. Saline washing is recommended to prevent any secondary infections to enter the ulcers and will also aid the healing process. Treatment is available to treat the symptoms, with the latest recommended treatments being found in the Clinical Effectiveness Guidelines (www.bashh.org; Pattman *et al.*, 2007).

Molluscum contagiosum

Aetiology

Molluscum contagiosum is caused by a pox virus and is a common skin infection particularly in children. However, it can be passed on during sexual activity to the genital area in adults. The virus is harmless and normally burns itself out in 12–18 months. In immunodepressant individuals, such as those who are HIV positive, the virus may take a lot longer with symptoms being more severe. It is, as its names suggests, very contagious and passed from one person to another via contact with the lesions.

Signs and symptoms

Molluscum is characterised by the appearance of smooth papules with an indented centre, which will heal on their own eventually. However, scarring may occur if punctured and secondary infections enter the lesions.

Diagnosis

Diagnosed on clinical appearance.

Treatment

As treatment may result in scarring, it is not normally recommended in children. However, treatment is available to treat the symptoms for those who have genital lesions, with the latest recommended treatments being found in the Clinical Effectiveness Guidelines (www.bashh.org; Pattman *et al.*, 2007).

Hepatides

Hepatitis is an inflammation of the liver and has a number of different causes: infection, other medical conditions, autoimmune disorders or alcohol abuse. This section will discuss the three main forms of viral hepatitis: A, B and C. There are also a number of others such as D, E, F and G but they are very rare. Each type attacks the liver and may even cause similar symptoms but the viruses are not related and offer no immunity against each other. Hepatitis is characterised by either acute or chronic.

Acute

This can have a sudden or gradual onset but is usually short lived, lasting only a couple of months resulting in only mild permanent liver damage. Rarely the acute stage can be fatal and can progress onto the chronic stage.

Chronic

This is subdivided into chronic persistent, which has a slow progression with mild symptoms but can develop into the second more severe form known as chronic acute. This can cause extensive liver damage, causing cirrhosis, liver damage and eventually proving fatal.

All viral hepatides are notifiable diseases and should be reported to Public Health and all sexual partners should be informed. See Partner Notification (Chapter 2).

Hepatitis A

Aetiology

Hepatitis A is caused by the virus HAV; it is tended to be thought of as the least harmful of the three viruses due to the normally mild symptoms and self-limiting nature of the virus. As with all the viral hepatides, it is extremely infectious. It is passed by ingestion from infected faeces and urine. The most common way is by eating food or drinking water that has been contaminated by HAV. An infected individual is at their most infectious before the appearance of symptoms, normally within the first 2 weeks of being infected. The virus can be found in semen, saliva and blood but not in high enough quantities to make transmission likely. Infection offers life-long immunity to HAV. There is a vaccine to prevent HAV.

Signs and symptoms
Often asymptomatic

- Flu-like symptoms
- Malaise
- Diarrhoea
- Fever
- Loss of appetite and weight loss
- Nausea and vomiting
- Upper right sided abdominal pain
- Generalised itching of the skin
- Jaundice – yellowing of the skin and whites of the eyes, dark urine and pale faeces.

Diagnosis
On positive serology.

Treatment
As such there is no treatment required, however, the current recommended management of the condition can be found in the Clinical Effectiveness Guidelines (www.bashh.org; Pattman *et al.*, 2007).

Hepatitis B

Aetiology
Hepatitis B is caused by the HBV virus and is usually mild with no long-lasting effects. However, a small number of individuals go on to have chronic HBV and remain infectious. Although they may have little or no symptoms, the virus will be attacking the liver resulting in permanent damage. It is normally passed via the sharing of needles or sexual contact by the passing of body fluids such as blood, semen and less likely saliva. On a positive note, there is a vaccine to prevent HBV.

Signs and symptoms
Often asymptomatic

- Flu-like symptoms
- Malaise
- Diarrhoea
- Fever
- Loss of appetite and weight loss
- Nausea and vomiting
- Upper right sided abdominal pain
- Generalised itching of the skin
- Jaundice – yellowing of the skin and whites of the eyes, dark urine and pale faeces.

Diagnosis
On positive serology.

Treatment
There is treatment available for those who are carriers. The current recommended treatment and management of the condition can be found in the Clinical Effectiveness Guidelines (www.bashh.org; THT, 2006).

Hepatitis C

Aetiology
Hepatitis C is caused by the HCV virus and is the most serious of the three hepatides. Most individuals do not clear the virus and a significant proportion can go on to suffer serious liver damage. It is passed on via infected blood through blood transfusion, infected needles used in piercing and tattoos or sharing of infected needles by drug users.

Signs and symptoms
Infected individuals can go on for many years with no symptoms at all but can include:

- Depression
- Confusion

- Tiredness
- Nausea.

Diagnosis
Positive Serology.

Treatment
There is treatment available for those who are infected by HCV but the liver damage can be so severe; it can result in a liver transplant. The current recommended treatment and management of the condition can be found in the Clinical Effectiveness Guidelines (www.bashh.org; THT, 2006). For Partner Notification see Chapter 2.

TAKING A SEXUAL HEALTH HISTORY

Taking an accurate sexual health history, along with Partner Notification, is one of the most important parts of the client pathway in a sexual health service. It is a specialist subject in its own right and most sexual health texts would devote a whole chapter to this subject on its own. (Wakely, 2003; Pattman *et al.*, 2005). However, since this is a text for those who are new to sexual health, it is unlikely you would be tasked with this role. But it is important to understand the importance and the basic principles of gaining an accurate sexual health history.

WHAT IS IT AND WHY DO WE NEED IT

A sexual health history is the gathering of information on the series of events preceding the client's current visit to the service and must be undertaken with a high degree of sensitivity. Issues such as confidentiality, being judged and concerns regarding their sexuality may all be barriers to obtaining an accurate sexual health history and therefore should only be undertaken by professionals who have received specific training for this role (Jolley, 2002).

SKILLS REQUIRED

Good communication skills – most important is to listen to the client. Many people find it hard to discuss the most intimate part of their lives to anyone, let alone a stranger, whom they have only just met and as such may not immediately get to the problem they are most concerned about. The use of standard forms where it is clear that everyone is being asked the same questions can contribute to the client feeling less intimidated and can act as a prompt for the health professional to ensure they have not forgotten anything. Watch as well as listen. Look at body language and remember it may have taken a great deal of courage to walk through a door which has the word 'sexual health service' written above it as this is a public admission of being sexually active.

Ensure the questions that are asked in a non-judgmental and non-threatening way and remember that individuals who are experiencing fear or embarrassment may mean the patient is not forthcoming in their information giving. Do not make any assumptions or interrupt the patient when they are giving you information. Imagine you are the client and address them as you would hope how you would be treated.

Health professionals should be able to justify their line of questioning. For example, asking what type of sex you have had would normally be unacceptable and intrusive but it is essential to discover whether they have had oral, vaginal or anal sex in order to establish which sites need to be sampled. Discovering how many partners, their partner's background such as country of origin (some parts of the world have higher incidence of infections than others), whether they are Intravenous Drug Users and whether they have practised safer sex will be needed to establish risk factors of whether they are at risk from certain infections such as HIV and hepatitis.

Another factor to remember is that if a client is presenting as a result of partner notification then coinfecting pathogens must be considered. Having one infection does not result in individuals being immune to others.

The environment is very important to obtaining an accurate sexual health history. A calm environment that is free from interruptions, such as phones ringing and other members of staff using it as a thoroughfare, will encourage an atmosphere of confidentiality. An explanation about the confidentiality policy of your service is important as clients may need reassuring as to who will see the information you are taking, what will be done with it and where will it be kept.

CONCLUSION

This chapter provided the reader with a basic knowledge base on the signs and symptoms of some of the more common SAIs, along with treatment regimes and an understanding of the basic principles of specimen collection and taking a sexual health history.

REFERENCES

British Association of Sexual Health and HIV(BASHH) Clinical Effectiveness Guidelines. www.bashh.org. Source: BMJ Publishing Group (www.stijournal.com).

Health Protection Agency (HPA) Diagnosis of selected STIs by country, English Strategic Health Authority, sex and age group, United Kingdom: 1997–2006. Available at www.hpa.org.uk

Jolley, S. (2002) Taking a sexual history: the role of the nurse. *Nursing Times*. Vol 98 (18):39–41.

Pattman, R., Snos, M., Handy, P., Sankar, N.K. and Elawad, B. (2005). *Oxford Handbook of Genitourinary Medicine, HIV and AIDS*. Oxford: Oxford University Press.

Public Health Laboratory Service (PHLS) (2002) *Investigation of Genital Tract and Associated Specimens*. London: PHLS.

Terence Higgins Trust (THT) (2006) *Sector Summary Report: Hepatitis A, B and C*. London: THT.

Wakley, G., Cunnion, M. and Chambers, R. (2003). *Inproving sexual health advice*. Radcliffe. London.

Wikipedia HIV (http://www.mcld.co.uk/hiv/?q=discovery%20of%20HIV).

Wikipedia Sexually Transmitted Disease (http://en.wikipedia.org/wiki/Sexually_transmitted_disease).

Wikipedia Virus (http://en.wikipedia.org/wiki/virus).

HIV/AIDS

4

Caroline Rowe

INTRODUCTION

Human immunodeficiency virus (HIV) is a communicable disease which is associated worldwide with poor health, decimation of specific communities, high treatment costs and care, significant death and poverty. The HIV epidemic has been around for about 25 years and at present a cure for HIV remains elusive. Developing drug therapies have ensured that people with HIV are living longer and experiencing an improved quality of life. For this reason, more and more experts are classifying HIV as a chronic condition rather than a life-threatening illness. This chapter will focus on HIV infection in adults. It will give an overview of the knowledge and skills required to test for HIV as well as detailing the natural history of HIV disease progression. HIV drug therapy will be reviewed and potential issues for people with HIV, around side effects of medication and adherence, will be discussed. Whilst the majority of preregistration nurses do not have direct responsibility for the nursing care of people with HIV, they have the potential to look after people with HIV on different placements. Therefore this chapter's aim is to increase awareness for preregistration nurses of some of the specific issues people with HIV have to face on a daily basis. For more information on the nursing competencies for people with HIV, review the National HIV Nursing Competencies (NHIVA, 2007).

LEARNING OUTCOMES

At the end of this chapter you will have:

❑ An increased knowledge and awareness of some of the specific issues people with HIV have to face on a daily basis
❑ An increased awareness of the natural history of HIV disease progression with specific reference to drug therapies
❑ Developed skills in the testing for HIV infection

BACKGROUND

HIV is a virus and like most viruses it needs a host cell in which to make more copies of itself in order for it to replicate and survive. HIV is classified as a retrovirus which is a ribonucleic acid (RNA) virus. Retroviruses have an enzyme called reverse transcriptase that gives them the unique ability of transcribing their RNA into deoxyribonucleic acid (DNA). The retroviral DNA can then integrate into the DNA of the host cell thus making the host cell an HIV factory. In humans, this host cell is part of the immune system and is known as a cluster of differentiation 4 (CD4) cell.

Healthy immune systems are able to deal with viruses, protecting the body from worsening disease or infections, however, because HIV attacks this immune system the normal process of protection ceases to work effectively. The role of the CD4 cell (also called the T helper cell) is to co-ordinate the immune system to fight off infection. Once the CD4 cells have been invaded by the HIV virus, they are not able to function normally resulting in a gradual decline in the immune system as more and more CD4 cells are destroyed.

If no antiretroviral treatment is commenced, the immune system becomes so depleted; it is not able to fight off infections or tumours that a normal healthy immune system would keep in abeyance. In HIV, these types of infections are called opportunistic infections and tumours as they take the opportunity to cause disease whilst the immune system is damaged. This is the time when a diagnosis of acquired immune deficiency syndrome (AIDS) can be made.

AIDS is a syndrome resulting from the damage caused by HIV. When a person with HIV is diagnosed as having AIDS, this means they have one or more of a defined list of otherwise usually rare illnesses as a result of the breakdown of the body's immune system. With the successful implementation of HIV drug therapy, fewer individuals with HIV go on develop AIDS. Once an AIDS diagnosis has been made, an individual life span will be limited.

EPIDEMIOLOGY

Although progress has been made in recent years to help combat the worldwide HIV/AIDS epidemic, the number of people infected with the HIV continues to grow year on year. In 2006, it was estimated that 40 million people were infected with the virus with around 3.8 million more people become infected with HIV yearly and 4.3 million dying of AIDS (UNAIDS, 2006).

In the United Kingdom, the HIV epidemic is relatively small with 63,500 (0.2% of the population) people living with HIV in 2005 (HPA, 2006). However, the impact of HIV has been substantial amongst certain groups, in particular the men who have sex with men community and, more recently, amongst people who have migrated to the United Kingdom from specific African countries. However, HIV can and does affect us all and anyone is at risk of contracting HIV if they carry out any high-risk behaviours.

Of those who have been infected with HIV in the United Kingdom up to 32% are unaware of their HIV status (HPA, 2006). In an attempt to try and reduce this number, the UK government through the Department of Health (DOH) (2001) set targets for all genito-urinary medicine (GUM) clinics to offer HIV test to all its new patients with a view to reducing the number of undiagnosed HIV infection by 50% by the end of 2007.

HIV TRANSMISSION

HIV is not a naturally occurring phenomena, it has to be transmitted from somewhere for an individual to become infected. Transmission of HIV occurs either through sexual contact, via blood or blood products or from mother to baby.

- Sexual contact – Most HIV infection is contracted through unprotected sexual intercourse. HIV is present in semen, pre-cum, vaginal fluids and menstrual blood. During unprotected sex with an infected partner, the HIV virus can transfer from one person to another through contact with the mucous membranes. As well as unprotected anal and vaginal sexual intercourse, HIV can also be transmitted through unprotected oral sex although evidence suggests this method carries less risk of infection. Certain factors will make the transmission of the HIV more likely, for example, if an individual has a pre-existing sexually acquired infection (SAI) such as chlamydia, they will be more susceptible to infection.

- Blood to blood contact – As HIV is present in blood, any contact with HIV infected blood has the potential to cause infection. The most common method of infection in this way is through the sharing of injecting equipment amongst injecting drug users. Infection with HIV is now very rare from blood transfusions because all blood which is donated for transfusion in the United Kingdom is tested for HIV and this has been done since 1985. Similarly all blood products such as Factor-VIII used to treat haemophiliacs are now heat treated to destroy any potential viruses. Infection through needle stick injuries is also very rare with less than 1% of individuals who receive injuries with HIV contaminated needles become infected.

- Mother to child transmission – HIV can be passed from mother to baby either before or during delivery or when breastfeeding. All pregnant women are offered and encouraged to have an HIV test because if HIV is confirmed during pregnancy, medication can be given to the mother to reduce the risk of HIV infection being transmitted to the foetus.

The risk of transmission also depends on the type of exposure and the infectiousness of the source patient. The risk of sexual transmission is estimated to be 0.2% (1 in 500) (Varghese *et al.*, 2002).

HIV TESTING AND SCREENING

The following information complies with best practice guidelines stated in the 'United Kingdom National Guidelines on HIV Testing 2006' (Rogstad *et al.*, 2006).

The only way in which HIV can be diagnosed is if an individual has an HIV test. Infection with HIV is most commonly diagnosed by a venous blood test, however, HIV tests can be carried out on saliva and blood spot test either in primary care settings such as specialist sexual health clinics or in secondary care through the GUM services. For best practice, it is recommend that all HIV tests are carried on blood as the evidence suggests the window period for HIV tests carried on oral fluid samples may be slightly longer (Rogstad *et al.*, 2006). All positive HIV tests need to be confirmed by a second sample taken at a different time before a definitive diagnosis can be given.

The blood test for HIV looks for antibodies to the virus rather than the virus itself. Antibodies are proteins produced by the immune system to fight specific bacteria, viruses or other antigens. Therefore, once the body has come into contact with HIV the immune system will start developing antibodies to fight off the infection. In the majority of individuals, it can take up to 3 months for these antibodies to be produced following infection with HIV. For this reason, it is recommended that HIV test are carried out 3 months after any HIV risk activity to rule out infection (Rogstad *et al.*, 2006). This is commonly known as the window period.

HIV test should only be undertaken with the person's specific informed verbal consent that should be documented (Rogstad *et al.*, 2006). This consent is often obtained during the 'pre-test discussion' which can be carried out by any appropriately trained healthcare professional. For HIV screening, informed verbal consent can be gained after the individual has read a patient information leaflet, however, it is essential to check that the individual understands the written information and that consent to HIV testing is obtained.

Pre-test discussion

Areas that need to be addressed in the pre-test discussion are:

- Knowledge of HIV infection and routes of transmission – Individuals can then assess their own risk as well as gain knowledge on risk reduction behaviours for the future.
- A risk assessment – If individuals are at high risk of HIV infection, they will require more in-depth pre-test discussion. This should be ideally carried out by someone, who has specific training and experience around HIV testing, for example, Sexual Health Advisers. It is important to establish

the date of last risk activity to ascertain if the individual is testing outside the window period. If the last risk activity has occurred within the last 3 months, an individual might need to return for another HIV test to confirm that the test result is negative. Apart from assessing potential sexual transmission of HIV, it is also important to assess other risk factors such as travel, drug use, occupation exposure and blood/blood products prior to 1985 (in the United Kingdom).

- History of previous HIV tests – This gives an indication of the individuals prior knowledge of HIV testing and if they have been able to reduce high-risk behaviour since the last test. It also indicates individuals who are having repeat HIV test because they are so fearful of HIV that they do not believe the previous negative HIV tests. These individuals should be referred on for further support and advice.

- Importance of testing – Testing enables individuals to be aware of their HIV status which allows them to make choices about their health. A positive HIV result allows individuals to be medically monitored and to commence drug therapy if appropriate. If individuals know they are positive, it also allows them to make informed choices around risk activities in the future.

- Implication of testing for mortgages, insurance, occupational risks and confidentiality – If individuals have an HIV test in a GUM clinic, they can be advised that their confidentiality will be respected according to common law, Sexually Transmitted Infections Regulations, Department of Health guidance, the Data Protection Act and the Regulating Body of the Health Care Worker, for example, Nursing and Midwifery Council. Individuals requesting a test should also be advised that having a negative result should not affect future insurance applications. A positive HIV result does affect an individual's ability to get mortgages and life insurance although it is not prohibitive.

- Giving the results – Individuals undergoing an HIV test need to be advised of how their result will be given. Results can be given in a variety of ways, for example, face to face, by text, by telephone and by post. The choice of method must be negotiated between the healthcare worker and the individual. If there is a strong possibility that the result will be positive, it is recommended that the results are given face to face and if possible by the same person who undertook the pre-test discussion.

- Explore future support – If there is a strong possibility that the individual will be HIV positive, it can be useful to explore how they think they would cope if the test was positive.
- Getting verbal consent for the test – This needs to be clearly documented in the individual's notes that consent has been given.
- Sexual Health Promotion – High-risk behaviours can be discussed and methods for their reduction can be explored, for example, safer sex.

More information on HIV testing can be found in the Manual for Sexual Health Advisers (SSHA, 2004).

Post-test discussion

Negative result
If possible, a post-test interview should be carried out as it can be useful to ascertain that the individual has understood the result and to ensure they tested outside of the window period so that the result can be confirmed. This can also be a good time to re-enforce sexual health promotion information on how to reduce future risk behaviour.

Positive result
The aims of this session are to ensure the individual has understood the result and answer any initial concerns and queries. Having a positive HIV test result can be very distressing; therefore, a psychological assessment should be undertaken. All positive results need to be confirmed by a separate sample; therefore, a further blood test needs to be carried out. Ongoing medical and psychological support needs to be negotiated and arranged. In general, this session is led by the needs of the person receiving the result.

Other areas that might be discussed include:

Partner Notification – Who else might be at risk of HIV infection? This is an issue that needs to be addressed, however, when an individual is potentially in shock following a positive diagnosis, this is often best followed up on subsequent visits.

Support – What support mechanisms does the individual have once they walk outside of the testing clinic. It can be useful to discuss what a newly diagnosed individual will do immediately after leaving the clinic and whom might they tell about their diagnosis, if to anyone.

As mentioned previously, 32% of people infected with HIV are unaware of their diagnosis. To try and reduce this number, all new individuals attending a sexual health clinic are offered an HIV test. This is called HIV screening. However, if an individual presents with any of the symptoms listed later, an HIV test is strongly recommended for diagnostic purposes.

CLINICAL FEATURES SUGGESTING HIV INFECTION
- Suspected primary infection with a seroconversion illness
- Any unusual manifestations of bacterial, fungal or viral disease: infection with tuberculosis; suspected *Pneumocystis jiroveci pneumonias* (PCP); or suspected cerebral toxoplasmosis
- Persistent genital ulceration
- Unusual tumours, for example, cerebral lymphoma, non-Hodgkin's lymphoma or Kaposi sarcoma
- Unexplained thrombocytopenia or lymphoma
- Unusual skin problems such as severe sebhorreic dermatitis, psoriasis or molluscum contagiosum, reoccurring herpes zoster or herpes zoster in a young person
- Persistent generalised lymphadenopathy (PGL) or unexplained lymphoedema
- Neurological problems including peripheral neuropathy or focal signs due to a space occupying intra-cerebral lesion
- Unexplained weight loss or diarrhoea, night sweats or pyrexia of unknown origin (Rogstad *et al.*, 2006).

STAGES OF HIV INFECTION
HIV disease progression is divided into four main stages. These stages, as written later, are for researchers and epidemiologists to be able to look at data surrounding HIV rather than an indication of an individual's medical condition where it is more pertinent to rely on blood monitoring and asking the individual

how they feel. Further information on HIV Stages of Infection can be found in '1993 Revised Classification System for HIV Infection and Expanded Surveillance Case Definition for AIDS Among Adolescents and Adults' (Centre for Disease Control, United States)

Stage 1 Primary infection
Stage 2 Asymptomatic infection
Stage 3 Symptomatic infection
Stage 4 AIDS

In the developing world, it is not also possible to rely on blood test to assist with medical monitoring, therefore the World Health Organization (WHO) has recently published the WHO Case Definitions of HIV for Surveillance and revised Clinical Staging and Immunological Classification of HIV-related disease in Adults and Children (2006 Revision) to facilitate HIV surveillance.

Primary
Individuals who are infected with HIV are often unaware that they have contracted the virus as they have no identifiable symptoms. Some people will have a short illness soon after they become infected – this is called a 'seroconversion illness' because it occurs just before the antibodies for HIV are produced in the body, when the HIV levels are highest in the circulating blood. It is at this point that infected individuals are most infectious.

Seroconversion
The symptoms for a seroconversion illness are vague and are often described as 'flu-like'. Symptoms typically begin 2–6 weeks post-infection with HIV and will last approximately 10–14 days.
    Symptoms can include:

- Fever and aching limbs
- Red blotchy rash over the trunk
- Sore throat (pharyngitis)
- Ulceration in the mouth or genitals
- Diarrhoea

- Severe headaches
- Aversion to light.

It has been estimated that up to 80% of people infected with HIV will develop some of these symptoms; however, because they are so vague and associated with other minor illnesses; they are not attributed to infection with HIV.

More rarely symptoms can include:

- Meningitis
- Paralysis
- Opportunistic infections.

If these rare symptoms do occur or if symptoms last longer than expected, then the prognosis for the individual is not so good. Without antiretroviral medication, it is likely that an AIDS diagnosis will be given within 5 years.

Asymptomatic

The asymptomatic infection stage is so called because people infected with HIV often display no visible signs of infection and disease progression at this point. This stage of HIV infection can last for many years.

If any symptoms are present, the majority of individuals will present with swollen lymph nodes, known as PGL. PGL is a sign that the body is attempting to fight off the HIV infection rather than a sign of any damage to the immune system.

Although individuals with HIV will have no visible signs of infection at this point, there is often damage to their immune system which is only detectable by specific blood tests. These blood tests include the CD4 count and viral load test.

Symptomatic

Research has shown that if left untreated, HIV will continually attack the hosts' immune system and cause more and more damage. The rate at which this damage occurs is very much dependent on the individuals' specific response to the virus. The more immunosupressed an individual becomes the more susceptible they are in developing infections and/or tumours indicating symptomatic HIV infection.

Specific action of HIV

The majority of symptoms seen in individuals with HIV are caused by the depletion of the immune function rather than the action of the virus itself. The only exceptions to this are HIV wasting syndrome and HIV dementia, which is caused by the direct action of HIV.

Opportunistic infections

Opportunistic infections are infections that a healthy immune system is able to keep under control, however, once the immune system becomes damaged from HIV; the infection takes the 'opportunity' to become a problem and cause ill health. The most commonly occurring HIV opportunistic infection in the United Kingdom is *Pneumocystis jiroveci (carinii) pneumonia.*

Tumours

Similarly, a healthy immune system is able to keep tumours and some cancers in abeyance, however, once the immune stops functioning effectively tumours and cancers can develop.

AIDS

AIDS is a diagnosis which is made only when certain medical criteria are met. For example, an individual with an AIDS diagnosis will have been diagnosed with an opportunistic condition such as PCP or Kaposi Sarcoma and have marked immunosuppresion.

MEDICAL MONITORING

Individuals infected with HIV and aware of their diagnosis require frequent medical monitoring for signs of immunosuppression. This is important because there is an optimum time to start HIV drug therapy. As well as clinical assessment monitoring of the immune function is undertaken through a variety of venous blood tests. The two most common tests are a CD4 cell count and a viral load test.

CD4 cell count

This blood test indicates when and if HIV is damaging the immune system. Doctors will look at CD4 cell count trends rather than one or two results as the CD4 cell count can go up and down due to many different factors, not just due to the effect of HIV on the immune function. For example, in women the CD4 cell count is affected by the menstrual cycle.

A healthy CD4 count will be within the range of 400–1600 cells/mm^3. Men on average have lower CD4 cell counts than women. Once infected with HIV, the CD4 cell count will drop and as HIV damages the immune system this decrease will continue.

Once the CD4 count drops to below 200 cells/mm^3, individuals are at risk of developing opportunistic infections such as PCP or tumours. To counteract this effect, people with HIV will be given treatment in advance to prevent them developing these opportunistic infections.

Viral load

This blood test indicates the amount of HIV in the circulating blood system. It is measured in the form of 'copies per millilitre of blood'. A low viral load test would be measured as 10,000 copies per ml and a high viral load test at 1,000,000 per ml. The aim of HIV drug therapy is to make the viral load test undetectable. This does not mean that HIV is eradicated from the body just that it is not evident in the circulating blood and or cannot be measured by current viral load tests as the amount of copies per ml is too low.

As with CD4 cell counts, viral load test are not seen in isolation. Doctors look for trends as the viral load can go up and down due to transient factors such as infection and following vaccinations.

PHARMACOLOGY

Since the availability of medication to combat the effects of HIV on the immune system in 1995, there has been a two-thirds reduction in the number of people dying from HIV/AIDS (Rogstad *et al.*, 2006). HIV drug therapy is known as highly active antiretroviral therapy (HAART) or antiretroviral therapy (ART).

The aim of HIV drug therapy is to reduce the amount of HIV present in the blood thus reducing the decline of CD4 cells resulting in a less damaged immune system.

There is an optimum time to start HARRT for individuals infected with HIV; however, deciding on the specific time can be a potential issue. Some researchers believe it is better to start treatment early when there is less damage to the immune system and more of a chance of getting the viral load to undetectable levels. Others believe that there is no proven evidence starting early provides any medical benefits. Once treatment is commenced, it needs to be taken regularly and correctly (see section on 'adherence') therefore starting too early puts more pressure on individuals to comply.

HIV drugs are never given in isolation. A combination of three or more drugs is always prescribed. Combinations are given in order to increase the likelihood of the therapy being able to prevent the replication of the HIV virus. This is achieved by the drugs inhibiting the HIV at different stages of its lifecycle.

Current classes of antiretroviral drugs

Nucleoside/nucleotide reverse transcriptase inhibitors

This was the first class of drugs available to treat HIV infection in 1987. Nucleoside/nucleotide reverse transcriptase inhibitors (NRTIs; also known as nucleoside analogues or nukes) interfere with the action of an HIV protein called reverse transcriptase, which the virus needs to make new copies. NRTIs are sometimes called the 'backbone' of combination therapy because most regimens contain at least two of these drugs. The advantages of NRTIs are that they have a low pill burden for patients with once daily options available and they have fewer drug induced side effects.

Non-nucleoside reverse transcriptase inhibitors

The second group of antiretroviral drugs approved in 1997 are the non-nucleoside reverse transcriptase inhibitors (NNRTIs). Similar to the NRTIs, NNRTIs (also known as non-nucleosides or non-nukes) stop HIV from replicating within cells by inhibiting the reverse transcriptase protein. Advantages of this class of drug are similar to the NRTIs.

Protease inhibitors

The third type of antiretrovirals is the protease inhibitor (PI) group. The first protease inhibitor was approved in 1995. Protease inhibitors inhibit protease, which is another protein involved in the HIV replication process.

Fusion or entry inhibitors

The fourth group of antiretrovirals is comprised of entry inhibitors, including fusion inhibitors. Entry inhibitors prevent HIV from entering human immune cells.

For further information on HIV medication, please review British HIV Association (BHIVA) Guidelines for the Treatment of HIV infected Adults with Antiretroviral therapy (Gazzard, 2006).

When to start drug therapy

The goal of anti-HIV treatment is to reduce the amount of HIV in the body. Certain criteria need to be met before treatment is recommended, however, any decision to start drug therapy is always a joint one between client and doctor. The combination of drugs an individual is prescribed is unique to that person in order to achieve the best possible potency, adherence and acceptability.

Prior to starting treatment, an assessment needs to be undertaken on the risk of the individual developing symptomatic HIV infection, if no treatment is started. This assessment is made looking at CD4 cell counts, viral load tests and physical examination.

Drug therapy is recommended before the CD4 cell count drops to 200 cells/mm^3 as at this level there is a strong possibility of the individual developing symptomatic HIV disease. Research has also shown that the drug therapy does not work so effectively when the immune system is so damaged. The majority of individuals with HIV commence therapy when their CD4 count is below 350 cells/mm^3.

ADHERENCE

The term adherence means taking medication exactly as prescribed, on time and following any diet restrictions. Adherence can be difficult and may require changes to an individual's lifestyle.

Nurses play a pivotal role in supporting individuals to adhere to their HAART regime. Research suggests (BHIVA, 2007) that brief one-to-one sessions focussing on patient treatment education with problem-solving skills increase adherence to HARRT in the short term. The HIV Nursing Competencies also highlights the importance of nurses supporting individuals with their therapy, working with the clients to develop a regime that is appropriate and relevant to them.

One of the most important factors for clients and doctors alike in deciding when to commence HAART is ensuring individuals are able to comply with the drug regime. It is important that anybody taking a course of medication takes it correctly to maximise the effect of the medication. However, with HIV, this is vital if the treatment is going to work effectively and not cause more long-term health problems.

The level of adherence needed for HAART is about 90–95%, considerably higher than most other medication. This is because HIV drugs have a short-shelf life in respect to keeping effective therapeutic drug levels high in the blood. It is therefore essential that people on HARRT do not miss doses because if they do HIV might continue to reproduce and as it replicates, it has the potential to develop drug-resistant strains. Drug-resistant strains of HIV are much harder to treat therefore increasing the likelihood of future treatment failure.

Adherence is influenced by many complex factors involving the individual with HIV, the regime they have to adhere to and the clinic prescribing their medication.

- Individuals have to be committed to starting the treatment regime
- Issues such as religious, cultural and health beliefs need to be explored before so that any potential barriers can be avoided
- A poor diet might affect treatments that need to be taken with food therefore a dietary assessment needs to be carried out and intervention instigated if appropriate
- Drug and alcohol use can affect the individuals ability to take medications on time
- Depression can affect the ability to take medication correctly
- The side effects of the drugs may prevent good adherence
- Being able to take medication when out and about.

Other factors which also need to be taken into account are the number of pills the individual with HIV has to take per day – this is known as the pill burden. HIV Nurse Specialist, Sexual Health Adviser and nurses are all in a position to offer help and support to people with high pill burdens thus making adherence more likely. It is important to ensure that the administration of the medication becomes part of the individual's normal regime rather than it taking over their lives. Drug companies produce many tools to help individuals with HIV with adherence. These include pill boxes, watches with timers and alarms, drug chats and single dose pill boxes.

The aim of successful drug treatment is to reduce the viral load of HIV in the blood to undetectable levels which in turn leads to an improvement in the immune function and halting the rate of disease progression resulting in improvements in quality of life for individuals with HIV.

If the viral load test becomes detectable again and the virus levels start to raise, it is a sign that this treatment regime has been unsuccessful. It is recommended that individuals switch to a new combination of drugs as quickly as possible if this occurs.

TREATMENT SIDE EFFECTS

Although substantial advances have been made in advancing HIV drug therapies, these medications do not come without side effects which have the potential to be more distressing for an individual than having HIV.

Treatment side effects are the effects a drug has on the body which are often expected outcomes. For example, when an individual initially takes ART, they can report feeling nauseous. This nausea is often short-lived, however, if it persists, steps can be taken to help relieve the symptoms.

Adverse drug reactions are those reactions which are not expected or predicted. The most serious of these seen is Stevens–Johnson Syndrome which causes blistering in the mouth and eyes and if left untreated can result in death.

Nurses play an important role in working with clients to monitor and report drug reactions and side effects. Reactions to a drug, which are not life-threatening, need to be weighed up against the effectiveness of the treatment. Often with support and advice, people with HIV can stay on medication and as their bodies get used to the effects of the drugs the side effects will diminish.

POST-EXPOSURE PROPHYLAXIS

Post-exposure prophylaxis (PEP) is a short-term antiretroviral treatment to reduce the likelihood of HIV infection after potential exposure, either occupationally or through sexual intercourse (PEPSI).

PEP is available to all healthcare workers who have a needle stick injury but is only recommended for those who are at high risk of HIV infection due to compliance issues with anti-HIV medication. For more information, review the following guidance 'HIV post-exposure prophylaxis: Guidance from the UK Chief Medical Officer's Expert Advisory Group on AIDS 2nd Ed, February 2004'.

The British Association of Sexual Health and HIV have produced guidelines on PEPSI – UK Guideline for the use of PEP for HIV following sexual exposure (Fisher, 2006).

PSYCHOSOCIAL ASPECTS OF HIV CARE

Although HIV has many physical symptoms associated with it, it can be the psychological, social and economic factors which have the most detrimental effect on an individual's well-being. The nursing care of people with HIV must therefore aim to provide an effective, appropriate and holistic approach to care with a view to maintaining an individual's quality of life. This can sometimes seem a difficult thing to achieve especially when in some communities HIV is still feared and HIV stigma and discrimination are rife. HIV stigma has been shown to have a detrimental effect on the well-being of individuals with HIV (Dodds, 2004) and for this reason, one of the aims of the National Strategy for Sexual Health and HIV (2001) in the United Kingdom was to tackle HIV stigma and discrimination.

STIGMA, DISCRIMINATION AND HIV

Stigma and discrimination are intertwined as stigma is the negative attitude towards a person with HIV, whereas discrimination is the act of doing something about it, for example, harassment, scapegoating and violence. Stigma and fear stop people talking openly about HIV in our society and therefore it prevents some people, who are at risk of HIV or fear they may have been infected, from seeking help, advice and support. Healthcare settings and personnel are not immune from displaying HIV stigma and discrimination due to fear and ignorance therefore it is essential that all trainee nurses have a good awareness of HIV Infection and challenge any stigma and discrimination they come across.

PSYCHOLOGICAL EFFECTS OF HIV

HIV is an incurable disease that has the potential to be life-threatening therefore people with HIV often experience detrimental psychological effects. Once someone has been diagnosed as HIV positive, their life will take a different path perhaps from the one they had planned or expected. People with HIV experience multiply losses such as loss of good health, loss of friends, loss of social status, loss of income and loss of predicted life expectancy.

During the progression of HIV, individuals will have to deal with specific issues with the first being coming to terms with their diagnosis. This can take many years as people with HIV need to come to terms with how they were infected, could they have prevented it, who can they safely tell about their status, whom do they need to tell as they might be at risk of infection and what will happen to them in the future. Coming to terms with an HIV diagnosis can for some individuals be similar to coming to terms with a diagnosis of cancer as described by Elizabeth Kubler–Ross (1969) in her grief cycle – denial and isolation, anger, acceptance, bargaining, depression and finally acceptance.

Later, in the progression of HIV individuals need to come to terms with ill health. For some, this means a loss of control over their body which can lead to a sense of having no control over their lives. HIV becomes the enemy and people with HIV report feeling persecuted by the virus (Schonnesson and Ross, 1999). Decisions about when to start therapy need to be made but will the therapy work, what to expect in terms of side effects, can adherence be maintained. Some individuals deal with this feeling of loss of control by being 'experts' on HIV, learning all about the virus, treatments and side effects of medications. This can be challenging for the multidisciplinary team caring for them but it does have the potential to foster a mutually satisfying therapeutic relationship between client and healthcare worker.

If an individual goes on to get an AIDS diagnosis, they then need to deal with the potential issues surrounding death and dying. It is at this point they might experience similar feelings they experienced when first diagnosed with HIV infection and go through the stages of coming to terms with dying as described by Kubler–Ross (1969).

Everyone with HIV is unique and their experience of dealing with HIV will be unique; therefore as nurses, it is essential to focus on the individual and how that individual experiences having an HIV diagnosis – appropriate specific holistic care.

HIV CRIMINALISATION

Over the past few years, there have been more and more cases documented of individuals being prosecuted for recklessly transmitting HIV infection to others. Any individual diagnosed with HIV needs to be aware of this fact and the steps they need to take to ensure they are not at risk of prosecution. These include advising all sexual partners of their HIV status before having any sexual intercourse and always giving correct information to sexual partners. Guidance around HIV criminalisation is changing all the time therefore it is recommended that any healthcare worker specialising in HIV keeps themselves up-to-date by accessing information from professional bodies such as NMC and organisations such as Terence Higgins Trust (THT).

The Crown Prostitution Services consulted with stakeholders on how best to proceed with alleged cases of reckless transmission of HIV and other SAIs. For an outline of their recommendations, see www.cps.gsi.gov.uk.

CONCLUSION

This chapter has given a brief overview of current HIV care and treatment. Twenty-five years on and the epidemic shows no signs of abating. Nurses are 'integral to the delivery of optimum care' to people with HIV (Weston, 2007). Preregistration nurses need to have knowledge and information about HIV so that they can appropriately care for people with HIV and perhaps become the next generation of nurses specialising in this speciality.

REFERENCES

British HIV Association (BHIVA) (2007), *Standards for HIV Clinical Care*, London: BHIVA.

Department of Health (DOH) (2001), National Strategy for Sexual Health and HIV. London.

Dodds, C. (2004), *Outsider Status Stigma and Discrimination Experienced by Gay Men and African People with HIV*, London: Sigma Research.

Fisher, M., Benn, P., Evans, B. *et al.* (2006), UK Guideline for the use of post-exposure prophylaxis for HIV following sexual exposure. *International Journal of STD and AIDS*, Vol 17:81–92.

Gazzard, B. (2006), British HIV Association (BHIVA) guidelines for the treatment of HIV infected adults with antiretroviral therapy, *HIV Medicine*. Vol 7: 487–503.

Health Protection Agency (HPA) (2006), *A Complex Picture: HIV and Other Sexually Transmitted Infections in the United Kingdom: 2006*, London: HPA.

Joint United Nations Programme on HIV/AIDS, UNAIDS (2006), *AIDS Epidemic Update: December 06*, Geneva.

Kubler-Ross, E. (1969), *On Death and Dying*, Macmillan Publishing, New York.

National HIV Nurses Association (NHIVA) (2007), *National HIV Nursing Competencies*, London: Mediscript.

Nilsson Schonnesson, L. and Ross, M.W. (1999), *Coping with HIV Infection: Psychological and Existential Responses in Gay Men*, New York: Plenum Press.

Rogstad, K.E., Palfreeman, A., Rooney, G., Hart, G., Lowbury, R., Mortimer, P., Carter, P., Jarrett, S., Stewart, E. and Summerside, J. (2006), British Medical Association. *United Kingdom National Guidelines on HIV Testing: Clinical Effectiveness Group British Association of Sexual Health and HIV (BASSH)*.

Varghese, B., Maher, J.E., Peterman, T.A., Branson, B.M., Steketee, R.W. (2002), Reducing the risk of sexual HIV transmission: quantifying the per-act risk for HIV on the basis of choice of partner, sex act, and condom use, *Sex Transm Dis*. Vol 29: 38–43.

Weston, A. (2007), cited in National Human Immunodeficiency Virus Nurses Association. National HIV Nursing Competencies London: Medicript Ltd.

USEFUL WEBSITES

Advice for Professionals on HIV/AIDS including Clinical Guidelines (http://www.bhiva.org).

British Association for Sexual Health and HIV (BASHH; http://www.bashh.org).

HIV Treatment Information (http://www.i-base.info).
Information and advice for people living with HIV/AIDS (http://www.aidsmap.com).
Information on HIV/AIDS (http://www.tht.org.uk).
Information on HIV/AIDS – Policies (http://www.dh.gov.uk).
Joint United Nations Programme on HIV/AIDS (http://unaids.org).
Medical Foundation for AIDS and Sexual Health – NHS HIV Standards (http://www.medfash.org.uk).
National HIV Nurses Association (http://www.nhivna.org).
Positive Nation Magazine (http://www.positivenation.co.uk).
Society of Sexual Health Advisers (http://www.ssha.info).
World Health Organization (WHO; http://www.who).

Contraception Including Emergency Contraception

5

Kathy French

INTRODUCTION

This chapter will provide up-to-date information on all methods of contraception available in the United Kingdom and provide background information on the evolution of each method. The legal status, efficacy rates, advantages, disadvantages, mode of action, contraindications, side effects, non-contraceptive benefits, if any, availability and the role of the nurse and others in the provision of each method will be addressed. The chapter will also address current training needs for nurses and provide useful links and websites for further information. After reading this chapter, the reader should be able to understand how the method works and be able to direct clients to appropriate services. Nurses and others wanting to work within contraception/sexual health services should be able to find suitable courses on the website www.guna.org.uk. This website has a list of courses available at post-registration level for nurses and advertises study days and conferences around contraception and sexual health. These courses are provided by the universities and may differ in content and number of credits allocated. Non-nurses can access excellent training courses from the fpa, formally the Family Planning Association, at www.fpa.org.

Work is currently underway to draft agreed recommended training standards for nurses at post-registration level in sexual health to ensure that the content and credits allocated to these courses are standardised throughout the United Kingdom.

It is not the aim of this chapter to provide the reader with the skills to prescribe, supply or administer contraception methods, but to provide up-to-date information to enable the reader to understand the various methods and also be able to signpost those needing contraception to appropriate services in a timely manner. Nurses who would like to specialise in contraception services would need to access a recognised course and these are available at the website www.guna.org.uk.

Up until the mid-1970s contraceptive methods were available from clinics but a nominal fee was levied for them and of course this fee may have been out of the reach of some members of the population. Organisations like the fpa and Brook played a key role in providing services for women and men. Since 1974, the availability of contraception has been free to men and women and this can only be seen as a positive health gain. Unfortunately, this is not the case in many parts of the world where such access to contraception is very poor and some women suffer the burden of additional pregnancies with the added risk to their health. Effective contraception would go some way in reducing the poor outcomes for women and their families. Contraception is highly effective, cost-effective and a health benefit to the population. Despite those benefits, contraceptive services are often the target of cuts. General practice provide around 80% of the provision, with community contraception services providing the remaining 20%; however, community contraception services provide 80% of the training needed to provide the service and therefore have a vital role in the future of the contraception. For every £1 spent on contraception services £11 is saved on health care (McGuire and Hughes, 1985).

In 2005, the National Institute for Health and Clinical Excellence (NICE) published their guide on long-acting reversible contraception (LARC); these methods include the intrauterine device (IUD), intrauterine system (IUS), sub-dermal implants and the injectable methods, in effect a method over 1 month's duration. The benefits of these methods include long duration and for some up to 10 years. Research by the fpa has shown that if women were informed about all methods, had a choice and access to LARC, this would reduce the failure rates of less reliable methods and more than that the National Health Service (NHS) in England alone could save some £33 million a year (Armstrong and Donaldson, 2005). A huge sum of money which almost amounts to half the cost of abortion services in 2003/2004 (Rosindell, 2005). In September, it was reported that women are still receiving inadequate advice on contraception (see www.contraceptivechoice.org.uk).

Hormonal and intrauterine methods of contraception became available in the 1960s, but the wider safer sex campaigns directed at blood-borne infection and sexually acquired infections (SAIs), including HIV (human immunodeficiency virus), did not go together with contraception, they were almost seen as separate entities. Despite the availability of condoms in one form or another, attitude towards their use, not just people's personal dislike of them, by some people are unfortunately widespread (Herring, 2003).

Although there are many methods of contraception available, some providers are unable for various reasons to offer all choice to women. As stated earlier, NICE LARC guidelines on long-acting reversible contraception key themes were to offer choice, better information and access and through clinical guidance and training of healthcare professionals. Long-acting methods are highly effective and less dependent on the user (NICE, 2005). Despite their known effectiveness, LARC uptake in the United Kingdom is very low accounting for around 8% of British women aged 16–49 years using them in 2003/2004 (Dawe and Rainsbury, 2003). A commentary in 2006 following the NICE LARC guideline concluded that the relatively higher initiation costs should not restrain the use of LARC as LARC results in greater cost savings compared to other reversible methods. They argue that LARC is not only effective but also a cost-effective option for the NHS (Mavranezouli and Wilkinson, 2006).

In terms of worldwide contraception use, maternal mortality is a rarity in the developed world, for example two deaths per 100,000 live births in Sweden whereas in the developing world, maternal morbidity and mortality is much more common. There are one or more maternal deaths for every 100 births in 17 of the 36 countries in West, Middle and East Africa (UNFPA, 2005). The benefits of contraception to these women would alter these dreadful statistics.

There are many myths about sexual health issues and contraception is no exception, for example some women have concerns about the dangers of the pill, mode of action of the emergency contraceptive pill and the IUD/IUS. Given the various pill scares in the media over the years, there is no wonder that some women continue to mention all the risks of the pill when trying to make a decision about a method, but may not be aware of the many benefits the pill offers. Some of the myths related to the pill are concerns that 'it may cause cancer,' 'increase weight' and can 'cause infertility'. These myths need to be dispeled. Some women highlight the problem a friend had when she stopped the pill, she took the pill for 5 years and when she stopped she could not conceive. It is important to remember that such woman may have difficulty conceiving regardless of contraception used and if they have never been pregnant in the past.

Research published in the *British Medical Journal* in 2007 stated that oral contraception in the UK cohort was not associated with an overall increased risk of cancer; indeed it may even produce a net public health gain. The balance of cancer risks and benefits, however, may vary internationally, depending on patterns of oral contraception usage and the incidence of different cancers (Hannaford *et al.*, 2007).

Guidance on methods of contraception derive from the United Kingdom Medical Eligibility Criteria (UKMEC) for contraceptive use and were adapted by the Faculty of Family Planning and Reproductive Health Care in 2006, this was adapted from the World Health Organization Medical Eligibility Criteria (WHOMEC). Clinicians prescribing any hormonal method of contraception should refer to the British National Formulary (BNF) and check the Faculty of Sexual and Reproductive Healthcare (FSRH) website.

Definitions of UK categories for use of hormonal contraception, IUDs and barrier methods are as follows, and clinicians will need to balance the benefits against the known risks when considering a contraceptive method for an individual woman. The UK eligibility criteria range from 1 to 4, with 1 having no restrictions for use, whereas 4 represents an unacceptable risk. These criteria form part of the decision-making process which a doctor or a nurse makes when helping a woman choose her method of contraception. It is important to remember that hormonal contraception is very safe, but existing medical history, family history and any medication may make it impossible for a woman to also use a specific method of contraception, for example having a first degree relative who had a stroke or heart attack at a young age or indeed the woman herself having had a deep venous thrombosis (DVT). The woman's lifestyle behaviour may also prevent the use of the combined oral contraceptive (COC) (i.e. smoking or obesity).

UK category	
1	A condition for which there is no restriction for the use of the contraceptive method
2	A condition where the advantage of using the method generally outweigh the theoretical or proven risks
3	A condition where the theoretical or proven risks outweigh the advantages of using the method
4	A condition which represents an unacceptable health risk if the contraceptive method is used

Health professionals advising women on contraception should inform them of all methods, including LARC, and these are outlined in the fpa leaflet which should be freely available in any service where women may ask about contraception. Methods which are part of the NICE LARC guideline will have LARC in brackets for ease of reading. Whatever method of contraception is chosen all women should be given written information about that method and the fpa leaflets are the preferred option, available from health promotion units. When counselling about contraception, the risk of an SAI should be part of the assessment as well. In September 2007, Talk Choice reported that research states that women are still not receiving comprehensive advice on contraception (see www.contracptivechoices.co.uk).

LEARNING OUTCOMES
By reading this chapter the reader will:

❑ Understand the mode of action of all contraceptive methods
❑ Be able to direct potential users to appropriate services
❑ Understand the benefits of emergency contraception

COMBINED ORAL CONTRACEPTIVE

In 1941, Marker used diosgenin from the Mexican yam as the raw material for sex steroids. The COC pill became available in the United States in June 1960 and in the United Kingdom in 1961 (Guillebaud, 2001, p, 97).

Current preparations of the COC pill contain two hormones, oestrogen and progesterone. Some preparations have a fixed dose of these two hormones; the dose is the same every day for the duration of the medication and is referred to as monophasic pills. Others have a phased dose with some variation in the amount of hormones used and are known as phasic pills. There is also an everyday (ED) pill which contains 21 active pills and 7 inactive pills (placebos); these are helpful for women who have difficulty remembering when to start a new packet. The COC is now widely accepted and available worldwide and became available in the United States in June 1960 and in the United Kingdom in 1961 (Guillebaud, 2001).

Efficacy rates

Methods of contraception can be judged to fail in two ways; one will depend on user failure and the other on method failure. Some methods are dependent on the motivation of the user, for example the condom, diaphragm, taking pills as per instruction and indeed attending for regular injections. All this might sound simple but for some this may prove difficult to fit in with the other pressures and commitments of daily living. On average, if 100 women are sexually active and do not use any contraception, some 80–90 of them will conceive in 1 year.

The COC is highly effective if used properly, that is, taken as per manufactures' instructions. This is a tall order for some women and they use various methods to ensure they comply with the instructions, for example some women take their pill at set times during the day and use modern technology to remind them, for example use of a mobile phone.

The fpa suggest that the COC is over 99% effective with consistent use (Guillebaud, 2001). The COC, however, does not protect against SAIs and the use of condoms is recommended as contra-infection.

It is important that woman requesting the COC should have an assessment as to their suitability for the method.

Mode of action

The COC provides blood levels of synthetic oestrogen and progestogen to prevent cyclical pituitary release of the follicle-stimulating hormone (FSH) and luteinising hormone (LH) which in turn inhibits ovulation.

Other actions include the thickening of the cervical mucus which reduces the ability of the sperm to penetrate. The COC also acts by thinning the endometrium (wall of the uterus) thus reducing the possibility of implantation.

All these actions are reversed once the woman stops the COC or if she regularly forgets the pill.

Legal status

Combined contraceptive pills are prescription only medicines (POMs) and need to be prescribed by a registered practitioner. Many nurses have undertaken Nurse Independent Prescribing (NIP) courses, whereas others may supply the COC using Patient Group Directions (PGDs)

Advantages

The COC offers highly effective contraception
Regulates the menstrual cycle
Protects against benign breast lumps
Reduces the incidence of dysmenorrhoea (painful periods)
Available from a variety of outlets
Does not interfere with sex.

Disadvantages

Increased risk of DVT/PE
Increased risk of blood pressure for some women
Does not protect against SAIs
Possible side effects initially including nausea, breast tenderness and mood changes.

Non-contraceptive benefits of the COC
Reduces the risk of ovarian, colon and endometrial cancer
Reduces the risk of benign breast lumps
Provides very good cycle control
May help with pre-menstrual syndrome (PMS).

Contraindications
Any contraindication to oestrogen, for example a history of DVT/PE
Raised blood pressure
Known or suspected pregnancy
Breastfeeding
Liver disease
History of migraine with aura
Very severe depression
Splenectomy for whatever reason
Any condition needing enzyme-inducing drugs which may alter the effect of the COC (i.e. epilepsy treatment)
Long-term immobilisation, for example leg in plaster.

When to start the COC
The COC can be started anytime in the cycle if the woman is sure she is not pregnant. Ideally, the woman should start the pill between day 1 and 5 of the menstrual cycle and will be protected against pregnancy immediately. Pills started after day 5 will not offer protection in that cycle and additional contraception will be needed. The COC is taken continuously for 21 days and then 7 days without pills which is often referred to as the pill free interval (PFI). In effect, 21 days with pills and 7 days without pills. It is during the PFI that the woman will experience a withdrawal bleed. Women who are prescribed antibiotics should be aware that these may interfere with the absorption of the pill. This is also true about other medications including those bought over the counter, for example St John's Wort, and women should be advised to inform the doctor/nurse of any medications whether prescribed or over the counter.

Missed pills (COC)
Women should be familiar with the guidelines for missed pills and the risk of a pregnancy developing will depend on the time the pill was missed and also the number missed.

Starting the new packet late or missing pill(s) at the end of the packet, in effect anything that lengthens the PFI poses a risk of pregnancy.

Number of missed pills (COC)	What to do?
Up to two pills anywhere in packet	Take the last pill missed immediately
	Take the remaining pills as usual
	Leave the earlier missed pill
	No additional contraception needed
	Take the last missed pill immediately
	Take the rest as usual
Three or more pills	Leave any earlier missed pills
	Use an additional method of contraception for 7 days
	Finally if the woman had unprotected sexual intercourse (UPSI) in the previous few days, emergency contraception (EC) may be indicated
	If seven or more pills left in packet, finish packet and have usual seven pill free days, but if less than seven, finish the packet and go straight to new packet without any PFI.

Availability
Combined oral contraception is available at community contraception clinics, general practice, gynaecology units, day surgery units and private abortion clinics.

Role of the nurse and others in the provision of the COC
Nurses are playing an increased role in the provision of the COC. Many have undertaken the NIP course and others have been trained in the use of PGDs. A PGD is a written instruction for the supply or administration of medicines to groups of patients who may not be individually identified before presentation for treatment. PGDs must be developed locally and involve the lead doctor, pharmacist and/or clinical governance lead for the Trust/Board. Models of good practice PGDs are available at the website www.portal.nelm.uk/pgd, these can be used as templates when PGDs are developed locally, they should only be downloaded and used as a template to meet local needs and

signed off by the relevant professionals. This allows greater access for clients in a variety of settings and has been one of the major advances for nursing in contraception/sexual health in the past 10 years.

Women often ask if they should take a break from the pill and the advice is that there are no known benefits from taking a break from the pill. A full medical and family history should be checked at subsequent visits to ensure there are no contra-indications to pill taking. It is important to be aware of the effects diarrhoea and vomiting may have on the pill, for example if sick within 2 hours of pill taking, this should be treated as a missed pill, a sit may not be absorbed. If diarrhoea continues for more than 24 hours, the same will apply. Some antibiotics affect the absorption of the pill and it is important that women are aware of this possibility. Women using the COC and complaining of breakthrough bleeding should be offered an SAI screen to exclude Chlamydia.

CASE STUDY

A 26–year-old woman attends clinic because she wants to go on the 'pill'. She smokes between 20 and 25 cigarettes a day and has a body mass index (BMI) of 31. She says her mother is taking high blood pressure pills and her father has diabetes.

She has tried to stop smoking but is not in her words 'too bothered'.

She thinks she would not want to use other methods of contraception; however, the doctor refused to prescribe the pill.

Reflection time

This scenario is fairly common in contraceptive services, mildly obese, smoking but also having a family history which is not ideal when using the COC. This young woman would be informed about the risk to her health from smoking, the need to reduce her weight and hopefully told about the benefits of exercise and calorie control. Any nurse or healthcare professional should be able to help her with that aspect of her life.

There are many things she can do to help reduce her chances of ill health later in life if she adopts a healthier lifestyle. She cannot,

> however, avoid the genetic predisposition to certain conditions but by making some changes herself will help reduce her chances of ill health later in life. She will need to be convinced of these in order to adopt the changes.
>
> She will not, however, be able to have the COC but can try the progestogen only pill (POP).
>
> Finally, it is recommended that the reader views the following website for any changes www.ffprhc.org.uk.

PROGESTOGEN ONLY PILL

Background to POP

The POP is only used by approximately 10% of women using oral contraceptives (Guillebaud, 2001). The POP is sometimes referred to as the mini pill as this is misleading as some women may think they are taking a mini version of the COC.

Mode of action

The main actions are in the thinning of the endometrium (lining of the uterus) and in some women ovulation may be inhibited in some cycles. Woman may be concerned that they are pregnant when they miss a period on the POP, but health professionals can reassure women that they are even better protected against pregnancy if they have amenorrhoea; however, a pregnancy should not be excluded either if a woman is new to the POP.

Legal status

Progestogen only pills are prescription only medicines and as such must be prescribed by a registered professional.

Efficacy rates

As with any medication which is dependent on the user, the POP is no different to any other medication. An overall rate of 0.3–4 per 100 women-years can be quoted with the higher rate occurring when the woman compliance is poor to the lower rate which applies especially to women who are breastfeeding (Guillebaud, 2001).

Advantages

No oestrogenic related side effects

Can be used for women who have contraindications to oestrogens, for example heavy smokers, raised blood pressure, previous history of DVT/PE, but who want to continue with an oral method of contraception

Does not interfere with breastfeeding

Good general tolerance of POP

Does not interfere with sexual act

Can be used at any age but useful for the older age group.

Disadvantages

The need to take the dose at the same time every day, has only a 3-hour margin if late taking the POP

Bleeding pattern may be altered with irregular bleeding

Possibility of functional ovarian cysts which may be painful

Higher risk of ectopic pregnancies if conception occurs, the POP does not cause ectopic pregnancies but does not protect against them

Does not protect against SAIs

Possible side effects when new to the POP, for example spotty skin, breast tenderness, weight gain.

Contraindications

There are fewer contraindications to the POP than to the COC and these can be found in the manufacturers' information sheets and are there for medico-legal reasons as there is limited epidemiological data to support them, and these include the following:

History of severe liver disease/cirrhosis/tumours

History of severe arterial wall disease

History of ectopic pregnancy

Undiagnosed vaginal bleeding

Known or suspected pregnancy

History of benign ovarian cysts

Current DVT/PE.

The POP may not be ideal for the very young who need to take the pill at regular intervals; however, a new POP was licensed in 2002, a desogestrel only pill called Cerazette. This pill has the added advantage of working like the COC by inhibiting ovulation but without the side effects of the COC and has fewer contraindications.

Cerazette should be started between days 1 and 5 of the cycle and it is taken in the same way as a COC and the woman has the same 12-hour window if she misses a pill. This is ideal for the young woman who prefers a pill but may not be good at remembering to take it at the same time every day. Cerazette is very effective against pregnancy offering less than 1% failure rate. The other advantage of Cerazette is related to the fact that ovulation is inhibited and therefore risk of ectopic pregnancy is unlikely. It is, however, more expensive than other POPs but being more effective should outweigh the initial cost.

When to start the POP

The POP can be started on any day of the cycle provided the woman is sure she is not pregnant but ideally between days 1 and 5 of the cycle.

It should then be taken at the same time every day and should be taken no more than 3 hours later from the chosen time every day. Missing the POP for more than 3 hours may put the woman at risk of a pregnancy and additional contraception or EC may be needed.

Missed pills (POP)

Missed pill	What to do?
Less than 3 hours late?	Take it immediately and continue as usual (If the POP is Cerazette the rules are different, it is 12 hours late, not 3)
More than 3 hours late?	Take pill immediately If more than one pill is missed, only take the last missed pill Take the next pill at the usual time, that could mean one is taken in the morning and another in the evening (two in 1 day) Continue in the usual way and use condoms or abstain from sex for 2 days

The POP differs from the COC in that the pills should be taken continuously without a break. It is also recommended that condoms are used as a contra-infection method.

CASE STUDY

A 19-year-old student is keen to go on the pill but she has contraindications to the COC. She is not keen to use other methods but also feels she may not be good at taking the POP at the same time each day. The decision was made to prescribe her Cerazette and she started with her next period.

Reflection time

This is an ideal method as there is no oestrogen in this pill, the young woman does not need to be tied to taking the pill at exactly the same time, she will be confident that she is well protected against pregnancy because ovulation will be inhibited. Time will need to be spent explaining how this pill differs from the other POPs in order for the woman to understand that she is using a POP but with the benefits of a COC.

INJECTABLE CONTRACEPTION (LARC)

Background to the method

It is estimated that some 40 million women worldwide have used long-acting contraceptive injectables with 25 million women currently using them, and many of these are in the developing world (Affandi, 2002).

There are two types of injectables, depot medroxyprogesterone acetate (DMPA) and norethisterone enanthate (NET EN). Depo-Provera is usually given as a three (3) monthly (12 weeks) dose of 150 mg. NET EN is recommended every 8 weeks as a dose of 200 mg. NET EN is licensed for short-term use only, for example to cover the period whilst a man is waiting for vasectomy results or if a woman needs short-term contraception.

DMPA has been recommended by the World Health Organization (WHO) and the International Planned Parenthood Federation (IPPF) and is available in many countries worldwide.

In 1984, the then Minister for Health recommended the suggestion by the Committee on the Safety of Medicines (CSM) that injectable contraception could be available for long-term contraception to women following counselling (Guillebaud, 2001).

Mode of action

Injectable methods of contraception have several actions; ovulation and ovarian production of oestradial are suppressed by inhibiting the secretion of pituitary gonadotrophins. The injectable also alters the composition and physical characteristics of the cervical mucus and the endometrium/lining of the womb. With prolonged use, the endometrium becomes atrophic and women may get amenorrhoea (stop having periods).

Depo-Provera appears to abolish peak levels of FSH and LH, but normal baseline levels are maintained during the period of medication.

Legal status

Injectable contraceptive methods of contraception are POMs and need to be prescribed by a doctor, nurse independent prescriber or can be administered by a nurse using a PGD.

Efficacy rates

Highly effective and limited margin for user failure. The range of efficacy for Depo-Provera is between 0% and 1% woman-years and for NET EN 0.4–2%. Pregnancy rates appear to be higher in the younger, more fertile woman and also for those women who are underweight.

Advantages

Very reliable method, invisible and provided the woman have regular doses, a pregnancy is unlikely.

Studies have shown failure rates ranging from 0 to 0.7 pregnancies per 100 woman-years (Lande, 1995).

Can be used by women who have a contraindication to oestrogen.

Does not interfere with breastfeeding.

Long duration (12 weeks) approximately four injections per year.

Benefit to women with history of heavy periods.

No storage needs, a benefit possibly for the younger woman who want to maintain their privacy around contraception.

Associated with less pelvic inflammatory disease (PID).

No ovulation pain.

Less growth of uterine fibroids.

Offers some protection against endometrial cancer.

Ideal for women who are unable to access services frequently.

Has a positive benefit for women with sickle cell anaemia as it is thought to bind the red cell haemoglobin and reduce the number of sickle cell crisis.

Disadvantages

Some women experience irregular bleeding initially but this generally settles after a few injections and some women experience amenorrhoea, this lack of periods can be a distinct advantage for some women, whereas others may prefer to have a regular monthly bleed.

Relatively long duration (12 weeks) if minor problems occur as the woman cannot stop the method.

Counselling is vital in order that women know the possible effects before they start the injection.

A small percentage of women may gain some weight on Depo and therefore a baseline weight is needed and if this does become an issue, the women may want to change her method. The weight gain usually happens in the first year and is thought to be due to an increased appetite.

There may be a delay in the return to fertility for some months and up to 18 months at the extreme end; however, some women may conceive very soon after stopping. These variations must be explained to women in advance.

Some women report depression, loss of libido, abdominal bloating, breast symptoms, all symptoms associated with progestogens.

Lack of periods may not be acceptable to some women.

Non-contraceptive benefits of the injectable

Reliable method against pregnancy and can be used by women who do not want their partner(s) knowing about their contraception. The woman does not need to rely on taking medication daily and is unrelated to sexual activity.

Benefits to women with a history of sickle cell anaemia as it binds the red cell haemoglobin and reduces the number of sickle cell crisis.

Long periods of amenorrhoea.

Some protection against cancer of the womb.

Contraindications

Concern has been expressed about the effect of Depo-Provera on peak bone mass. Bone mass is a major determinant of skeletal strength and there is a wide variation in bone mass between races. For example, Caucasians on the whole have lower bone mass than black people and Asians have lower bone mass than Caucasians. Peak bone mass is also dependent on nutrition, exercise, hormonal status, genetic factors and by any disease altering factors. Evidence suggests that oestrogens are crucially important in attaining peak bone mass in women (Woolf, 1998). With the suppression of ovarian function and low levels of oestrogen amongst some women, concern has been expressed about the long-term use of Depo-Provera. Several studies have looked at the effects of long-term use of Depo-Provera and results are mixed.

With these mixed results and the knowledge that if there is a reduction in the peak bone mass on Depo-Provera, these effects are reversible once the method is stopped, similar to what occurs during long periods of breastfeeding. It would be unfortunate that women would be deprived from a reliable method of contraception.

The key points of the prescribing authority are the following:

- In adolescence, Depo-Provera may be used as first-line contraception but only after other methods have been discussed with the patient and considered to be unsuitable or unacceptable.
- In women of all ages, careful re-evaluation of the risks and benefits of treatment should be carried out in those who wish to continue the use for more than 2 years.
- In women with significant lifestyle and/or medical risk factors for osteoporosis, other methods of contraception should be considered.

This advice is compatible with the guidance from the Faculty of Family Planning and Reproductive Health Care Clinical Effectiveness Unit (CEU) Guidance on 'Contraception choices for young people' (October 2004) which states that 'for some young women, injectable methods, which avoid reliance on daily pill-taking, may be preferred'.

In terms of counselling women about Depo-Provera, the woman should be informed about the long-term effects together with an assessment of her lifestyle choices about diet, exercise, alcohol and smoking habits. With the limited evidence available, women who have a poor diet, smoke and drink more than the recommended units of alcohol, who are very unfit or who are on long-term steroids should be advised to consider an alternative method of contraception.

It is not considered necessary to measure oestradiol levels during medication unless there is a concern about a fracture risk after some years of use. There is no need for a woman to have a bone scan before starting the injection.

When to start the method

Both methods should be given between day 1 and 5 of a normal menstrual cycle and it is important to take a good sexual health history to exclude a possible pregnancy.

It can be given immediately following an abortion or miscarriage but is best to delay the first injection until at least 21 days following a delivery regardless whether the woman is breast-feeding or not. The sooner the injection is started after delivery the more likely the woman will experience heavy prolonged bleeding and with a new baby she does not need this additional problem and also she may stop sooner. It can be given immediately following an abortion carried out in the first and second trimester and/or miscarriage. It is also recommended that condoms should be used as a contra-infection method.

Route of injection

The injection should be given deep intra-muscular in the buttock. It is important that the whole dose is given otherwise efficacy rates may be affected. The injection site should not be massaged afterwards as that increases the absorption. The site selected and whether right or left should be recorded in the medical notes, this is important because an infection or abscess could develop unrelated to the injection site and if any doubt existed a further injection may be needed. This would be extremely rare indeed but one where efficacy could be affected.

Check latest BNF for list of drug interactions.

Missed injection

The injection is licensed for 12 weeks and 5 days; therefore, the woman should be advised to return for a repeat injection every 12 weeks. Some women may choose to have the injection sooner if, for example, they are going on holiday and it is not unusual for a woman to have an injection early at around 10 or 11 weeks.

If a woman misses the injection she can have it up to 14 weeks, but it is important to ensure that she is not pregnant and a careful history must be taken.

CASE STUDY

A 25-year-old woman who is a smoker and has a BMI of 20 is requesting the injection. Whilst taking a sexual health history she tells you her mother who is 57 years has been told she has 'thinning of the bones'.

Both mother and daughter smoke and have a reasonable amount of alcohol each week. It was difficult to judge the daily diet of this young woman but she did admit that she does not do any regular exercises. Following counselling the young woman decided to try another method of contraception. In this case it is not the injection which is dangerous but the lifestyle of the user and future risks to her health could be prevented by switching her method of contraception. She may continue to smoke and not exercise but any health problems will not be related to the injection.

Reflection time

Although this woman was keen to use the injection, it is the responsibility of the prescriber to alert/inform her of the known risks as well as the benefits to any method. The woman cannot expect the doctor or nurse to prescribe her a medication which might adversely affect her long-term health, especially when other methods are available.

SUB-DERMAL IMPLANTS (LARC)

Background

The first sub-dermal implant available in the United Kingdom was Norplant, with six rods.

Norplant is no longer available in the United Kingdom and has been superseded by Implanon® which is the only sub-dermal implant available.

Implanon®, containing the progestogenic hormone etonogestrel is a single 49 mm rod some 2 mm in diameter and about the size of a matchstick. The implant is much easier to insert and remove than Norplant and is licensed for 3 years.

Mode of action

The hormone etonogestrel 68 mg is released in a controlled manner over a period of 3 years and acts in the same way as the injectable method by inhibiting ovulation, thickening the cervical mucus which in turn prevents sperm penetration and causes thinning of the endometrium.

LEGAL STATUS

The sub-dermal contraceptive implant is a POM and licensed for 3 years.

Efficacy rates

The sub-dermal contraceptive implant is conservatively described as being over 99% effective against pregnancy.

Advantages

Effective method lasting 3 years and very convenient

Long action without need for change and no concern about 'missed pills'

Does not interfere with the sexual act

Steady blood levels rather than fluctuating levels

Oestrogen free and can be used by women with contraindications to oestrogen

Speedy reversal and return to fertility once removed

No effect on blood pressure

Invisible to others

Provides a constant level of hormones
Reduced risk of ectopic pregnancy
Is easily inserted by the trained professional.

Disadvantages
Irregular bleeding pattern for some women
Possible local effect, for example discomfort at insertion and removal
It is a minor procedure needing an experienced professional
Possible local trauma
Minor side effects may continue until implant is removed
Some women may experience mood swings, acne, weight gain and loss of libido (rare)
Not suitable for women using enzyme-inducing drugs.

Contraindications
Progesterone dependent tumours
Severe liver disease
Known or suspected pregnancy
Acute porphyria
Sensitivity to any component.

Non-contraceptive benefits
May offer some protection against cancer of the womb

Insertion techniques
The implant is inserted in the under section of the upper less dominant arm. Local anaesthesia is used to reduce the pain and the implant is inserted by using the self-loaded implant from the sterile pack. The implant will be palpable with the fingers once inserted.

Timing of Implanon® insertion
Ideally, the implant should be inserted between day 1 and 5 of a woman's natural cycle. It is advisable to use additional contraception for 7 days if inserted on or after day 5. It can also be inserted immediately after a first trimester abortion and around day 21 after a pregnancy or a second trimester abortion.

Implanon® can be inserted at any time if the woman is using the COC or the injectable and either continues with previous method or use condoms for 7 days after insertion.

No specific follow up is necessary but women should be advised to return to any clinic if concerned. She should also be given the date/time of removal and re-insertion (3 years). Implanon® is radio-translucent and if the implant is not palpable, it can be removed with the aid of ultrasound.

Role of the nurse and training issues

Since December 2003, Implanon® and local anaesthetic needed have been included in the BNF. Nurses have been inserting implants for some time with the support of medical colleagues who hold a Letter of Competency (LoC) from the FSRH. Some 600 nurses have been accredited by the Royal College of Nursing (RCN) to insert contraceptive implants and they can also train other nurses following the criteria laid down by the RCN guideline for nurses to fit sub-dermal implants (discussed later).

Many nurses are currently trained and accredited to insert sub-dermal implants and the RCN holds a database of these nurses for England, Scotland, Wales and Northern Ireland.

It is also recommended that condoms should be used for contra-infection.

CASE SCENARIO

An 18-year-old student attends the clinic requesting a reliable method of contraception. She has used condoms in the past but now has a regular boyfriend who is going to university with her. She has regular periods and no contraindications to any method of contraception.

She is keen to try the implant and feels this would be ideal as she could forget about it for 3 years. She returns when she gets her next period between day 1 and 5 for the insertion.

She appears pleased that whilst at university she does not need to worry about contraception and she is aware of SAI risk and will use condoms.

This is an ideal method for a young woman about to embark on a degree because she may not have access to all methods of contraception locally and she does not have to attend clinics at regular intervals.

> **Reflection time**
>
> What are the key benefits of sub-dermal implants?
>
> The surgery/clinic is not keen for younger woman to have this method because of the initial cost.
>
> How might you argue for a change of opinion about this?
>
> Initial cost should not be the factor.
>
> Very effective method could help reduce the teenage pregnancy rates and abortion rates and this in turn reduce the overall health budget.
>
> It is important to approach this not simply from the stance of 'my service cost' only but the wider NHS costs and more importantly for the woman concerned.

CONTRACEPTIVE PATCH

Background

Patches have been used in many areas of health care, for example for women taking hormone replacement therapy (HRT) and for those trying to give up smoking and where nicorette patches are used.

Evra was and still is the first hormonal contraception method presented in a transdermal delivery system. The patch contains norelgestromin and ethinyloestradiol and in effect is like a weekly dose of the COC in a patch delivered transdermally. The patch is a thin beige three-layer matrix type and sticks to the skin like a plaster and is $4.5\,cm^2$.

Mode of action

It acts in the same way as the COC, but releases a daily dose of the hormones through the skin into the blood stream for 7 days.

Legal status

The contraceptive patch is a POM.

Advantages

The advantages are the same as for the COC but additionally do not have to be taken daily.

Is unrelated to the sexual act

As it is absorbed through the skin, it does not cause any gastric upsets

Reduces the need for daily pills
Easily reversed
Gives good cycle control like the COC.

Disadvantages
The same as the COC.

Can fall off and women need to be told what to do if this
   happens
The patch has good sticking properties and should be placed on
   buttocks, back or inner arm but not the breasts, upper abdomen or face.

Non-contraceptive benefits
May reduce the risk of fibroids, ovarian cysts and breast disease
   (not breast cancer)
May protect against the risk of cancer of the ovary, womb and
   colon.

How to use/when
The patch can be applied anytime in the cycle provided the
woman is sure she is not pregnant but ideally started between
day 1 and 5 of the normal cycle and this will offer immediate
protection against pregnancy. The patch is changed 7 days later
and then every 7 days for 2 weeks – a total of 21 days of patch
use plus 1 week without a patch.

Patch for 7 days, day 8 changes to new patch, day 15 change
to new patch and then 7 patch free days.

What if the patch falls off?
The patch has good sticking properties and should be placed on
buttocks, abdomen, the back or upper arm but not on the chest
or breasts. Daily activities like swimming, showering and exercise do not appear to affect the adherence of the patch to the skin
even in hot or warm temperatures. If for some reason (rare) the
patch does come off the fpa offer the following suggestions:

- If the patch has been off for less than 24 hours no additional
  contraception is required.

- If it has been off for longer than 48 hours then another method of contraception is needed for the next 7 days and EC should be considered (fpa, 2003).

A protective label is provided for the disposal of a used patch as it should not be flushed in the toilet in case some of the hormone remains in the patch.

Condoms should be recommended for contra-infection.

CASE STUDY

Fiona a 25-year-old woman wants to change from the COC which offers her very good cycle control and less heavy periods. She says she does not have period pains anymore but due to work and frequent travel she worries about missing a pill. Other methods were explained to her and the patch appealed, she was prescribed it and informed about how and when to change the patch. She reported back in 3 months and said she was very happy with the method and no changes to report and her concern about missed pills were addressed.

Reflection time

What benefit might this method have over the COC?

Ideal for the woman who may want the benefits of the COC but who has difficulty remembering a pill every day.

Should the cost be a factor?

INTRAUTERINE CONTRACEPTION (LARC)

Background

The first mention of the intrauterine contraception device was by Hippocrates (c. 460). Over the centuries various materials have been used for IUDs including glass, pewter, ebony, gold and wool. All of these at some point in history have been thought to prevent pregnancy and needless to say, not without severe risks to the woman, in previous generations women like now have tried to prevent pregnancy and accepted the possible risks which were part of that decision. In 1909, Richter developed a ring-shaped device made of silkworm; Grafenburg modified this by covering it with silver wire (Guillebaud, 2001) and this was known as the Grafenburg ring.

Plastic was used for the first time in the production of an IUD in the 1960s and the Lippes Loop and the Safe-T device became the IUD of choice. Some women experienced heavy bleeding and period pains with these devices and smaller plastic devices containing copper were developed and these reduced the side effects and also increased the efficacy rates. Some midwives prefer to abbreviate the IUD to IUCD arguing that in obstetrics an IUD is an intrauterine death but the agreed abbreviation and the commonly understood term is IUD and will be referred to as such in this section. The word 'coil' should be avoided as this conjures up endless images of wires and loops in the minds of women and indeed some professionals. Although the IUD is safe and effective against pregnancy, it is estimated that only 5% of women aged 16–49 years currently use an IUD (FFPRHC, 2002).

Mode of action

The primary mode of action is the prevention of fertilisation due to direct toxicity and an inflammatory reaction within the endometrium may have an anti-implantation effect should fertilisation occur but the IUD is not an abortifacient (FFPRHC, 2004). The number of sperm reaching the Fallopian tubes is reduced, sperm motility is disrupted and the ova development impeded (Dennis and Hampton, 2002). It is believed that IUDs containing copper have a toxic effect on both sperm and ova which renders their survival unlikely. Alterations in the copper content of cervical mucus may also inhibit sperm penetration of ova (FFPRHC, 2002)

Legal status

IUDs are medical devices and do not need to be prescribed.

Efficacy rates

The copper-releasing IUD is an effective method of contraception.

Women should be advised of the low failure rate generally around 1% and efficacy rates will depend on three key factors:

(1) The skill of the professional fitting the device.
(2) The type of the device, the more copper in the device the lower the pregnancy risk.
(3) The risk of expulsion without the woman's knowledge.

There are few systematic reviews of randomised control trials (RCTs) that allow direct comparison of pregnancy rates with different devices (FFPRHC, 2004). The WHO states that an IUD is a very effective method with 0.6–0.8 pregnancies per 100 women in the first 12 months and women are advised that the failure rate is 1%. This needs to be explained to women that for every 100 IUDs fitted a year, one woman will become pregnant.

Advantages of the IUD

Very effective and effective immediately after insertion
Lasts between 3 and 10 years, the IUD with the longest licence should be used to prevent risk of infection at time of removal and refitting
Can be used as an emergency method of contraception
No user failure rate
Does not affect future fertility, return will be immediate after removal
Does not interfere with sexual act.

Disadvantages

Does not protect against an SAI
Is an invasive procedure
Needs specific training for the healthcare professional in order to gain the skills of fitting an IUD
Possibility of heavier and more painful periods for some women in the first 3–6 months of use
Small risk of pelvic infection within the first 20 days after insertion
Can lead to expulsion without the woman knowing
Small risk of perforation through the womb at time of fitting or later.

Contraindications of fitting an IUD

Pregnancy or suspected pregnancy
Undiagnosed vaginal bleeding
Allergy to copper (rare)
Post-partum sepsis
Current history of PID or SAI or within the past 3 months
Distorted uterine cavity
Women with cervical cancer
Women with known pelvic TB
Ovarian cancer
Past history of bacterial endocarditis
Menorrhagia (the IUS would be the method of choice)
Following delivery of a baby – the device should be deferred until after 4 weeks post-partum
Vaginal discharge which may be caused by a sexually transmitted infection.

Counselling before fitting an IUD

Women should be informed about all methods of contraception and that the IUD will not protect against an SAI and therefore condom use is advisable as well. An explanation of the failure rates and what to do if a pregnancy occurs must be given to the woman. An SAI risk assessment should be made and if a risk exists, the woman and her partner should be offered screening and treatment before a devise is fitted. The younger the woman and the more sexual partners she has, the greater her risk of PID. Prophylactic antibiotics are not recommended for routine IUD fitting unless there is a risk of an SAI and subsequent PID.

Risk of expulsion (1 in 20) should be explained and is more common in the first 3 months after insertion.

Perforation at time of fitting or immediately afterwards occurs in about 1 in 1000 insertions and this needs to be explained.

Fitting of IUDS

IUDs must be fitted by a doctor or nurse who has been trained specifically in the technique, for doctors guidelines are available from the FSRH and for nurses and midwives, the RCN have guidelines based on the training for doctors (listed later).

An IUD may be fitted within 5 days of the earliest expected ovulation or at any time in the cycle provided that there is no possibility of an existing pregnancy. An IUD can also be fitted immediately following a first and second trimester abortion and after 4 weeks post-delivery. A fitting should be delayed after a caesarean section, see www.ffprhc.org.uk/publications.

Women should be offered a chaperone during the procedure in case of an emergency and emergency equipment must be available in all settings where IUDs are inserted. The procedure is done using a 'non-touch' technique.

Follow-up care

Once the device is fitted, the woman should return to clinic after her next period or 3–6 weeks after insertion of the IUD. Women should be advised to return at anytime if concerned or has any abnormal pain or bleeding otherwise no need to be seen until removal/change of device. The IUD can be removed at anytime in the cycle provided another device is inserted, but if failure to insert a new device, additional methods must be used.

Occasionally, the device may be expelled either with the woman's knowledge or without and it is important that she is told how to check the threads of the IUD at regular intervals. If she suspects or a health professional suspects the device has been expelled, an ultrasound scan needs to be performed to confirm or otherwise the presence of the device. Additional contraception must be used until the results of the scan are known.

If the device is located within the uterine cavity, it can be left there until it is due for replacement and the woman reassured it is still effective despite the missing threads. Of course a pregnancy needs to be excluded whilst this is investigated.

If a woman does get pregnant with the device *in situ*, she can be advised that there is no evidence for any increased risk to the developing foetus. The woman should be advised to seek advice as there is an increasing risk of miscarriage with an IUD *in situ*. The position of the device can be located by the use of an ultrasound and generally the device is below the sac and easily removed by an experienced person. If the device is above the sac it is considered unwise to remove it as this may interfere with the sac. The risk of miscarriage is thought to be in the region of 50% (Guillebaud, 2001). This should be dealt with by an experienced doctor.

If an IUD remains *in situ* during the pregnancy it is important to remove this at the time of delivery, otherwise the woman may not be aware that she still has the device and some time later does not understand (nor do the professionals) why she is having difficulty conceiving.

Nurses and IUDs

In some parts of the world nurses and midwives insert IUDs as part of their role; however, this did not happen in the United Kingdom until the 1970s and even then only in very few centres. One of the first centres which allowed nurses to train in the technique was Kings College Hospital in London. Nurses were trained by lead consultants and senior doctors and they were the pioneers. During the late 1990s and early 2000s more and more nurses extended their role in contraception/sexual health and this came about because nurses were generally extending their scope and the service delivery was changing with many roles traditionally performed by doctors being done by nurses. Many nurses have now been trained and accredited by the RCN and are training other nurses to take on this procedure in both general practice and within contraception/sexual health services. A study undertaken in 1999 compared the expulsion rates and follow-up needs between doctors and clinical nurse specialists (CNS) at Kings College Hospital in London where these CNS had been fitting IUDs since the mid-1970s and there was no difference between the two groups (Andrews *et al.*, 1999).

As stated earlier IUDs should only be fitted by doctors and nurses who have followed the recommend training laid down by the Faculty of Family Planning and Reproductive Health Care for doctors and RCN guidelines for nurses.

Condoms should also be recommended as a contra-infection method.

IUDs as an emergency method of contraception

An IUD can be inserted as an emergency method of contraception and should be offered to all women who request an emergency method. The advantage of the IUD is twofold, one it can be inserted up to 5 days post-UPSI and can be the ongoing method of contraception with long duration. The counselling, information, fitting procedure is as per IUD. Additionally, the woman may be at risk of an SAI and antibiotics may be given at the same time and screening for SAIs done. This is a balance between the risk of a pregnancy and a possible risk of an SAI which can be treated in prophylactic way.

CASE SCENARIO

A 27-year-old woman stopped the COC 4 months ago when her relationship ended. She met with her ex-boyfriend last week and they had UPSI 4 days ago. She had not thought that she could be at risk of a pregnancy until she confided in a friend. Her friend advised her to get the 'emergency pill'. It was now some 90 hours since UPSI and the offer of an emergency IUD was recommended. The woman decided to have the IUD fitted and would consider this as an ongoing method of contraception. Risk of an SAI was also discussed and she felt she was not at risk as neither she nor her partner had any other partners since the separation. She returned 3 weeks later saying she had decided to continue with the method and was seeing her partner again.

Reflection time

A woman is requesting EC but is too late for EC (hormonal) method; however, she concerned that this is an abortive agent.

How might you help her understand how the IUD works?

Could you explain to her why it should not be fitted if the woman is already pregnant?

Would you know where to refer her?

INTRAUTERINE SYSTEM (LARC)

Background

The levonorgestrel-releasing intrauterine system (LNG-IUS) releases $20\,\mu g$ of the hormone into the uterine cavity through its polydimethylsiloxane reservoir. The only system in current use is the Mirena.

Legal status

The IUS (Mirena) is a POM and is licensed for 5 years, it is not, however, licensed for EC. The IUS should not be referred to as a coil or a device, it is a system. Nurses who are not nurse independent prescribers will need a PGD in place.

Mode of action
The main mode of action is via local hormonal effects in the uterine cavity, prevention of endometrial growth, alteration and thickening of the cervical mucus and uterotubal fluid which impair sperm migration and inhibit sperm motility and function. The blood levels are less than that observed in women using the POP. The majority of women will continue to ovulate while using the IUS despite some women not having periods.

Efficacy rates
Efficacy rates with the IUS are very good, around 0.2 per 1000 woman-years and are effective for 5 years.

Advantages
Effective method of contraception

Last 5 years

Reduces heavy bleeding and this can be a major advantage for women with high iron deficiency anaemia

Return to fertility is rapid

Convenient

Few side effects

Not depend on woman having to remember to take daily pill

Reduced period pains

Can offer protogenic protection for woman using oestrogen replacement therapy

Risk reduction in extrauterine pregnancies (ectopic pregnancies)

Can be used during breastfeeding.

Disadvantages
Possible higher rates of bleeding in the early months of use (up to 6 months)

If a pregnancy occurs (rare) the risk to the developing foetus is unknown

A major disadvantage in developing countries may be the cost as the system is much more costlier than a copper device.

Non-contraceptive benefits of the IUS

Can be used by women who are taking HRT

Effective for the treatment of heavy bleeding.

Contraindications

Known or suspected pregnancy

Presence or recent SAI

Unexplained uterine bleeding

Allergy to the system

Distorted uterine cavity

Active liver disease

Previous attack of bacterial endocarditis or presence of heart valves

Not licensed for EC.

Fitting the IUS

Same procedure as the IUD.

Nurses and the IUS

Nurses who are trained to insert the IUD should also be competent to insert the IUS; RCN accreditation is not possible without being competent various of IUDs including the IUS.

CASE STUDY

A 31-year-old woman is keen to use the IUD, she has a regular partner and has completed her family. Following a sexual health history she mentions that her periods have been heavier over the past 2 years since she had her last baby. Her current method of contraception is the diaphragm, but she says she often forgets to use it and does not want another pregnancy. You inform her about the benefits of the IUS which she has never heard of and she decides to try the method. She returns to clinic for the fitting 1 week later when she has a period. She has the IUS fitted and reports back some months later when she has cervical screening that she is delighted with the method and her periods are so much lighter. A successful method for that individual woman.

Reflection time

A woman is about to embark on HRT for early onset of the menopause but she needs contraception as well; how might you link this up for her in terms of the IUS?

Could you explain the dual role?

DIAPHRAGMS AND CERVICAL CAPS

Background

Before the discovery of hormonal and intrauterine contraception, female barrier methods (diaphragms and cervical caps) were common methods of contraception used by one in eight couples in the United Kingdom. Female barrier methods are effective in preventing pregnancy if used consistently and properly, but the effectiveness against SAIs is limited (FFPRHC, 2007). They are very ancient methods dating back to 1850 BC; the Petri papyrus describes a spermicidal pessary made party of crocodile dung (Guillebaud, 2001).

Mention is made of the use the tops of lemons and limes (shape similar to modern diaphragms) during medieval times. The tops of the fruit were used to cover the cervix and the acid juice was believed to destroy the sperm and possibly any risk of infection. Whether this is true or not, one cannot be sure but without doubt women throughout history tried various things to prevent an unintended pregnancy.

With the development of rubber caps and diaphragms became popular in the 1920s and were heralded as the salvation for women who would be in control of their fertility. Despite the innovation in rubber devices, these were not independent of intercourse and not as effective as the methods we have today but paved the way for better methods for couples.

Diaphragms and cervical caps come in various sizes and every woman must be individually fitted with the correct size and this is done by a vaginal examination by a competent health professional. Women will need time to practice the skill before they can rely upon the method and patience is needed to ensure the woman understands how and why to fit and remove. Women should be given the patient information leaflet for recommended duration of use for specific diaphragms and cervical caps.

Legal status

Diaphragms and caps are medical devices.

Mode of action

Diaphragms and caps act as barriers to sperm entering the cervical canal and therefore need to be fitted initially by a professional skilled in the procedure. As hormonal and other methods of contraception have developed, the use of diaphragms and caps have declined.

Advantages
Offers protection from SAIs but not considered to be adequate protection against HIV and viruses
Considered more natural by some
No hormonal effects
Woman in control of method and only use when woman has sex
Does not affect breastfeeding
Fairly effective against pregnancy if used properly
Cheap and only need to use with intercourse.

Disadvantages
Needs to be fitted properly and reliant on user motivation
As spermicidal creams are recommended, can be perceived as messy
Not independent of the sexual act
Can be fitted incorrectly
Some women sensitive to the rubber and spermicidal cream/jelly
Some women complain of frequent cystitis when using this method
May not fit well if increase or decrease in weight of more than 7 lb.

Non-contraceptive benefits
Protection against SAI
Reduces the risk of cervical cancer.

Efficacy rates
The most quoted overall failure rate is around 2–20 per 100 woman-years with the lower rate amongst the older experienced women. Failure rate will depend on several things, was the device fitted properly, was it used in a random manner or not at all and/or was it removed too soon after intercourse? Women often choose this method for spacing the family and maybe when a pregnancy might not be a problem.

Fitting

As stated earlier these should be fitted by a competent healthcare professional initially and the women given time to practice the procedure before she relies upon the method. The use of plastic models can be very helpful to help women understand where the cervix lies in relation to the vagina. Whether a diaphragm or a cervical cap is fitted, it should be correctly fitted for each individual woman and contraceptive clinics will have experienced staff who has the skill to fit them properly. Women who are not familiar with the use of tampons may need additional support in fitting.

FSRH recommend that women using barrier contraception should be aware of EC in case the device becomes dislodged or removed too soon and they also support the advance supply of hormonal EC.

CASE STUDY

A 38-year-old woman with a regular partner wants to stop taking the COP; she is very fit and active and has no health problems. She has a busy lifestyle, her family are complete and she wants to try the diaphragm. The nurse arranges the fitting and she is able to fit it herself very easily. The nurse advises her of the benefits of the device and that she needs to have it checked every 6 months or sooner if she has a change in her weight for any reason. She said she was increasingly fed up with daily pill taking and wanted something without hormones. When she returns in three months she reports that she has lost four pounds and the nurse checks the device and it still fits well, the woman is very happy with the method she feels 'better' not taking hormones anymore.

Reflection time

You are the nurse in the clinic and had limited knowledge of caps or diaphragms and a woman asks if you could supply her one.

Would you be able to tell her how it works and the benefits of the method?

Could you be able to signpost her to a clinic or surgery locally where staff are trained to fit them?

STERILISATION – FEMALE AND MALE

Female sterilisation

Female sterilisation is a widely used modern method of contraception in the world and is achieved by the blocking of the uterine tubes (Fallopian tubes) in order to prevent the transport of the ovum to the uterine cavity and this is achieved by cutting the tube, applying clips or rings.

Laparoscopic sterilisation is a common gynaecological procedure in the United Kingdom and should be seen as a permanent procedure and only agreed to be provided when no more pregnancies are planned. Counselling is important as the couple may not be aware of the permanency of the procedure and there are very good alternative long-acting reversible methods of contraception available, for example the IUS, sub-dermal implants and both of these methods may have added benefits for the older women. Many women seeking sterilisation and who have used one method of contraception happily all their reproductive life may not be well informed about LARC. Evidence suggests that a significant number of women have regrets about having a sterilisation and up to one-third of them seek reversal later (Hills *et al.*, 1999). Reversal is a costly procedure and may not be generally funded by the NHS.

There is no need in law for the partner to sign the consent form for the woman requesting the procedure; however, the decision to proceed with sterilisation should be from both parties.

Efficacy rates

The overall failure rate with female sterilisation is about 1 in 200, but if done using a special clip known as the Filshe clip the failure rate in 10 years after the procedure may be lower in the range of 1 in 333–500 women (fpa, 2007).

Male sterilisation or vasectomy

Male sterilisation is called vasectomy and with the use of local anaesthetic the tubes (vas deferens) are cut and stitched to prevent sperm travelling into the penis. The incision is very small and takes place in the scrutum. Dissolvable sutures are used and ongoing contraception is needed until two consecutive negative sperm counts are provided.

Advantages of sterilisation
No further need for contraception
Does not interfere with sexual act
Removes the fear of another pregnancy.

Disadvantages
Does not offer any protection against infections (SAIs)
Difficult to reverse and costly
Rarely done on the NHS
May be regretted
Family circumstances may change and more children desired
Sperm may be present for several months following vasectomy

There is no evidence that either sterilisation or vasectomy will affect the libido.

LACTATIONAL AMENORRHEA METHOD
Occasionally professionals will be asked about the 'breastfeeding' method?

It is important that professionals understand that such a method does exist and is known as lactational amenorrhoea method (LAM). This is not a recognised or recommended method but some women may ask about it.

Whilst it has been known for some time that breastfeeding can delay the return to fertility, the conditions under which women could reliably take advantage of this were not fully understood. In 1988, scientists meeting in Bellagio, Italy proposed how postpartum women could use LAM as a contraceptive method. They concluded that women not using contraception must be:

(a) fully or nearly fully breastfeeding
(b) not having periods (amenorrhoea)
(c) no more than 6 months post-delivery.

Women who fit into these three criteria had less than 2% chance of conceiving (www.linkageproject.com).

Breastfeeding delays the resumption of normal ovarian cycles by disrupting the pattern of female hormones.

Women in developed countries may need to rediscover this method and may resume bottle-feeding their babies sooner than women in developing countries that have discovered this benefit of breastfeeding. The woman must fit into the three criteria above to be protected and if in doubt a reliable method which does not affect the breast milk should be advocated. Professionals must not say if you breast fed your baby you will not get pregnant and advice woman about a more reliable method of contraception.

CONDOMS

There are two types of condoms one male and one female. Regardless of the method of contraception condoms should also be used to reduce the risk of an SAI/HIV and HPV (human papilloma virus), this is referred to as the Double-Dutch method.

MALE CONDOM

Condoms have been with us for a long time and are thought to have been invented by a Dr Condom, a physician to Charles 11 but as Guillebaud says it is doubtful whether Dr Condom ever existed (Guillebaud, 2001). Whatever the origin of condoms in the past were linen sheaths moistened with lotions to prevent venereal diseases. Some condoms were made from animal bladders. In 1844, Hancock and Goodyear were responsible for the vulcanisation of rubber and in turn revolutionised barrier contraceptives. Condoms have suffered from poor press and many users argue that they interfere with the sexual act. It remains a sad fact that the broadcasting companies are still unable to advertise a condom outside the packet and yet sex is portrayed on the TV all the time.

It is important to consider the role condoms have in the prevention of both SAIs and HIV, these are all preventable conditions and whilst many young people focus on pregnancy prevention, some are still reluctant to use a conta-infection method. Any effort to reduce the risk of SAIs and HIV should include the promotion of condom use; otherwise the effort will be ineffective. It is estimated that a minimum of 8 billion condoms would have been needed in 2000 in order to achieve the kind of access required for significant reductions in the rate of infection and prevalence in the developing world and Eastern Europe (Population Action, 2002). The challenge to condom use for some people is lack of availability and whilst condoms are free from community contraceptive services and GU clinics, many general practices fail to supply them. In order to raise awareness of condoms, the Department of Health launched a campaign in December 2006 titled 'condom-essential wear' which aimed to promote condoms almost like any other item, for example a mobile phone. Until it becomes 'uncool' to have sex without a condom, some young people will continue to place themselves at risk. Media images of people having sex without a condom do little to promote the use.

Effectiveness of the male condom
It is very difficult to measure failure rates with condoms but two randomised trials included in a Cochrane Review investigated breakage and slippage rates as part of longer contraceptive efficacy studies (FFPRHC, 2007). That said the true failure rate of male condoms in the first year of use is approximately 2% but can be as high as 15% and this will depend on many variables, for example experience of user, type of condom and the use of any lubricant. Oil-based lubricants like baby oil, sun cream or massage oil should not come in contact with condoms otherwise these will destroy the rubber and render them ineffective.

Condoms should be encouraged amongst all sexually active people and their use normalised; however, prospective users need to be shown how to use them properly. Without the familiarity of how a condom is fitted and if sex takes place in a hurry with a new partner, there is a recipe for disaster waiting to happen.

Condoms are for a single episode of intercourse and a new one used each time.

Advantages of male condoms
Protects against pregnancy
Protects against SAIs
Protects against HIV
Protects against cervical cancer in women
Reduces the risk of PID.

Disadvantages of male condoms

Needs motivation to use

Needs the knowledge and skill to use competently

Not freely available for all you need them.

FEMALE CONDOM

The female condom has been available in the United Kingdom since 1992.

The female condom is made of polyurethane rubber and the rim fits around the cervix offering protection against pregnancy and SAIs, however it has not been widely accepted by users. One of the disadvantages of the female condom is that it can allow penetration between the condom and the vagina as it does not fit well. Women complain that it is similar to a crisp bag in terms of noise.

Effectiveness of the female condom

If used according to instructions it is about 95% effective.

Advantages of female condoms

Reasonably effective if used correctly

Can be used with another method

Are contra-infection as well as contraceptive

Does not interfere with breastfeeding

Can add to the fun of love making

May be seen as more natural by some

Readily available from many outlets

No medical side effects.

Disadvantages of female condoms

Reliant upon user motivation, skill and knowledge

Can be seen as messy

Embarrassing for some to suggest use in advance of sex

Does interfere with sexual act.

Condoms should be part of all consultations on safer sex practices, regardless of the sexual orientation of the client group. School-based sex education sessions could normalise the use of condoms and challenge some of the myths surrounding their use. Young girls are often reluctant to raise the issue and some young men are not equipped with the skill to use them. Condoms are frequently missing from TV advertisements for fear of upsetting viewers and yet the benefits from using them are many.

Contrary to common belief, HIV interventions which include information on condoms do not inadvertently encourage an earlier sexual debut, more frequent sexual partners or more sexual partners according to a meta-analysis of 174 studies reported in 2006 (Edwin, 2006).

FERTILITY AWARENESS/NATURAL FAMILY PLANNING

Fertility awareness is based on working out the safest time in a woman's cycle to have sex to avoid an unintended pregnancy. In order to calculate the 'safe period' a woman should define the shortest and longest menstrual cycle over at least the previous six cycles (Guillebaud, 2001).

If 100 sexually active women do not use any contraception, some 80–90 of them will become pregnant in a year. The menstrual cycle will vary between woman and even at different times in the life of an individual woman but generally the cycle is around 28 days long but regardless of the length of the cycle ovulation will occur around 10–16 days before the start of the next period.

The first infertile phase starts on day 1 of the cycle and ends with the earliest time that sperm could survive to cause a pregnancy. This will depend on the follicular response to the pituitary hormones and this can vary enormously during a woman's life time. Women considering this method of contraception should seek the expert advice of a healthcare professional skilled in the teaching of fertility awareness. The method may be very acceptable for those couples who have religious objections to 'unnatural' or hormonal methods of contraception. One of the advantages of this method is once taught and understood woman have a greater understanding of their cycle and no further expense or follow up is necessary and it has the added benefit that once couples understand the cycle it can be used to achieve a pregnancy. For further information on fertility awareness/natural family planning see www.fertilityuk.org

PERSONA

A device called Persona® is available from chemists which was marketed in 1996, this is a disposable test using sticks which are placed in a hand-held computerised monitor. The sticks are dipped in an early morning urine sample and hormone levels are measured and once the significant levels of hormones are detected, the woman enters into the 'unsafe' period of her cycle. This is denoted by a green light changing to red. Couples need to be aware that the failure rate is about 6% which is 1 in every 17 chance of a pregnancy in a year. Another important issue is the use of Persona following the use of EC; the woman must wait for 3 months before she resumes reliance on Persona. This product is not available in contraception clinics.

NEW METHODS

The arrival of a vaginal delivery ring is expected later in 2008. The ring will be a flexible, transparent and almost colourless ring which will deliver two hormones, etonogestrel and ethinyloestradiol over a period of 3 weeks. In effect the ring will be similar to a low dose combined pill but the advantage will be the woman will not need to remember a pill every day.

It is difficult to say anything more about this new additional advancement in contraception but any option which makes the lives of women easier must be welcomed.

EMERGENCY CONTRACEPTION

Introduction

The section will focus on the important matter of EC, the historical background, efficacy rates, modes of action and how an assessment is made about the need for EC. At the end of this section the reader should have a good knowledge of the method, understand when to take it in terms of efficacy rates, know about both methods and be able to direct/signpost those needing EC to the right place at the right time. Some nurses should be able to supply EC using a PGD.

There are two methods of EC, the hormonal method and the emergency copper bearing IUD. The IUS is not licensed for EC. Any woman seeking EC should be offered both methods.

Learning outcomes

After reading this section the reader should be able to:

- Understand the mode of action of both the methods of EC
- The importance of a good sexual history to calculate the need for EC
- the importance of SAI screening

Emergency hormonal contraception

EC provides women with a safe means of preventing a pregnancy and is used following UPSI. Women throughout history used various methods, including douching, honey, garlic, fennel, elephant dung and Coca-Cola to name a few.

The Persian physician Al-Razi suggested: 'first immediately after ejaculation let the two come apart and let the woman arise roughly, sneeze and blow her nose several times and call out in a loud voice. She should jump violently backwards seven to nine times'. Jumping backwards supposedly dislodged the semen, whereas jumping forwards would assure a pregnancy (Guillebaud, 2001).

The more effective methods began in 1963 at Yale University in the United States and in the mid-1970s a Canadian gynaecologist devised the combined hormonal emergency contraceptive. The combined oestrogen and progestogen method of EC was licensed as PC4 in 1982 and often referred to as the Yuzpe regime. The method which contained ethinyloestradiol 50 mg (times 2) and levonorgestrel 250 mg (times 2) was the only hormonal emergency method available. Whilst this regime prevented many pregnancies it also had to be taken 12 hours apart, had some minor side effects and was contraindicated in women who could not take oestrogen.

Other studies discovered that pregnancy could be prevented by the use of progestogen only formulations, known as POEC. This was a major advance because the combined method was often contraindicated for some women in the same way as the COC might be. In a large multi-centre Random Controlled Trial (RCT) in 1998 by the WHO reported in the Lancet demonstrated that progestogen only emergency contraception (POEC) was more effective, had fewer side effects and had fewer contraindications and was licensed in 2000 as Levonelle-2®.

On 1 November 2005 Levonelle 1500® (one tablet) became available as a POM in the United Kingdom. Prior to that it was available as two tablets each containing 750 µg and was taken together as one single dose, a major advance for women. Levonelle 1500® must not be confused with Mifespristone which is prescribed for medical abortion as Levonelle 1500® and Levonelle One Stop® are not abortive agents and known or suspected pregnancy prohibits their use. In 2002, a Judicial Review rules that pregnancy begins at implantation and not at fertilisation, thus EC is not considered an abortifacient (DH, 2002).

It is often argued that having EC more widely available would increase risk-taking amongst women and would also adversely affect their use of regular contraceptive methods. Reported evidence demonstrates otherwise as stated in a recent publication (Trussell and Guthrie, 2007). Health professionals providing EC in non-clinical settings should work to locally agreed clinical pathways and most recent guidelines ensuring women get optimum device and treatment.

Mode of action

The exact mode of action is not fully understood but it is believed to inhibit ovulation rather than inhibit implantation. When given before the LH surge when the follicles are less than 15 mm in size follicular rupture was prevented or ovulatory dysfunction was apparent. If taken prior to ovulation EC can inhibit ovulation for some 5–7 days by which time any sperm in the upper reproductive tract will have lost their fertilising ability (FFPRHC, 2006).

Legal status POM and P

Levonelle 1500® is a prescription only medication (POM) and Levonelle One Stop® is a pharmacy (P) medication. The pharmacy medication is available from the pharmacist has a cost attached to it, currently around £25 whilst it is free from community contraception clinic and general practice; however, many woman opt to pay the fee for convenience and to prevent a pregnancy and one needs to welcome this additional choice for women.

Effectiveness of EC

EC, either Levonelle 1500® or Levonelle One Stop® should be taken within 72 hours of UPSI but the sooner the better. It is not licensed for use after 72 hours but if given between 73 and 120 hours women should be advised about the limited evidence of efficacy and an IUD would be the preferred method. A large study by the WHO provided evidence that LNG continues to reduce the expected pregnancy rate if taken between 73 and 120 hours after UPSI but as stated above this remains outside the product licence (FFPRHC, 2006).

Of the pregnancies that could be expected if no EC had been used the EC will prevent:

- Up to 95% if taken within 24 hours
- Up to 85% if taken between 25 and 48 hours
- Up to 58% if taken between 49 and 72 hours (fpa leaflet).

If there is any doubt about whether a woman should have EC or not, it is best to give it provided she is not pregnant.

Advantages

Effective at preventing a pregnancy if given as soon as possible after UPSI

Available widely from a variety of outlets, Brook, contraceptive/ sexual health clinics/A&E departments/walk-in centres/school nursing services/some gynaecology units and pharmacies

Safe with very few side effects

One-off tablet.

Disadvantages

Need to access services to get it

Need to know the time limits (72 hours)

Does not protect against an SAI.

Contraindications

It is important to understand that despite the myths often expressed, EC *per se* carry almost no health risk no matter how often used but at certain times in the cycle or if delayed they are less effective (Trussell and Guthrie, 2007).

When to take EC

EC should be taken as soon as possible after UPSI and no later than 72 hours. The earlier the better and the WHO state that each 12 hours delay raises the risk of pregnancy by almost 50%, for example taking EC within 12 hours of UPSI is more effective than taking it at 48 hours post-UPSI and 48 hours is better than 60 hours.

Before starting EC the health professional must take a careful sexual health history, including date of last menstrual period, whether this was normal and ask about any other episodes of UPSI in this cycle. This is very important as some women may not consider a previous episode of UPSI important or which may pose a risk of pregnancy. If there is any chance that a pregnancy has occurred then EC is contraindicated.

An assessment should also be made about the risk of an SAI and screening offered later. See Chapter 3 on incubation period and screening too soon may give a false negative result. Ongoing contraception needs to be discussed and all options offered to the woman.

EC and the use of liver enzyme-inducing drugs

The Faculty of Family Planning and Reproductive Health Care Clinical Effectiveness Unit published a guideline recommending that women who are using an enzyme-inducing drug, for example Griseofulvin, Carbamazepine, Rifampicin, and others (see BNF) who require EC should increase the dose of EC by 100%. The CEU advises that women should take the initial dose as soon as possible after UPSI and repeat the dose 12 hours later. There is no data available on side effects and that this is outside the product licence.

Follow-up advice

The woman should be advised to return to the provider if she misses the next period, has any unusual bleeding or sudden abdominal pain. She should be advised that her period may be early, on time or delayed by a few days, this will depend on the individual woman.

EC should not be relied upon for ongoing contraception.

The role of the nurse and pharmacist

There has been many changes in the availability of EC over the past 10 years. Nurses and pharmacists can supply EC by the use of a PGD and many nurses can also prescribe it. Pharmacists can provide it over the counter medication. This is a major advantage for nurses working in a variety of settings, for example within the school setting, A&E departments and walk-in centres as they can provide EC to women easily.

Nurses who are not able to prescribe should ensure they have a PGD in place, written by the lead doctor, pharmacist and/or clinical governance lead. A PGD template for Levonelle® is available at www.rc.org.uk/publications and at www.ffprhc. org.uk.

CASE STUDY

Kerry, a 20-year-old woman requests EC having had UPSI some 24 hours ago. She ran out of the COC 2 weeks ago. It is Saturday evening and her local clinic is closed but a friend told her she can access this via her pharmacy. Her last normal period was 10 days ago and potentially she is at risk of a pregnancy. She attends the pharmacist and after counselling the pharmacist advises her about the method and discusses ongoing methods. She is given Levonelle One Stop® and takes it as instructed and returns to her regular clinic the following week to get another supply of COC and an unintended pregnancy was avoided.

Intrauterine EC

When a woman requests EC it is vital that the health professional, whether doctor, nurse or pharmacist takes an accurate history around date of last period and whether the period was normal. This is vital because the woman could already be pregnant and taking EC will not prevent that pregnancy ongoing and fitting an IUD would be a criminal offence knowing the woman was pregnant as it could cause an abortion. It is also important to ask if other episodes of UPSI took place as some women may not mention this in the real belief that they were not at risk then. It may be too late to commence hormonal EC and women may be able to have an emergency IUD.

An IUD, any copper bearing device can be fitted up to 5 days after UPSI or up to day 19 of a 28-day cycle. This must be calculated carefully as fitting an IUD knowing or suspecting a woman is pregnant is in effect procuring an abortion.

An emergency copper bearing IUD is more effective than EHC and has the advantage of being used as an ongoing method of contraception. Fitting of the IUD is the same as fitting at any other time but it may be necessary to provide prophylactic antibiotics at the same time as screening for SAIs would not be able to provide results if the method is being fitted as an emergency.

The IUS is not licensed for EC.

CASE STUDY

A 17-year-old woman requests EC as she had UPSI 32 hours ago with her regular partner. She was using the COC but missed two pills as she went away for the weekend. The nurse assessed the risk for pregnancy with her and offered her both methods of EC; she opted for the hormonal method, as she was very happy with COC. She resumed the COC immediately.

Reflection time

Would you be able to talk to a young person through EC, the time limits and how it works?

Would you know which clinic/service to send her to for help?

Do you know what pharmacy provision there is in your area/ locality?

Would you be able to supply EC (hormonal) by the use of a PGD?

If yes, would you be able to know how to go about getting a PGD written?

Would you known where to refer a woman for an emergency IUD?

Conclusion

This chapter provided an overview of all methods of contraception, included information on PGDs and provided useful websites to direct the reader for additional information. EC, covering hormonal and intrauterine, was also addressed. Some references relate to the Faculty of Family Planning and Reproductive Health Care and others to the FSRH. The organisation changed their name in 2007.

REFERENCES

Affandi, B. (2002), Injectable contraceptioives: A worldwide perspective, *The Journal of Family Planning and Reproductive Health Care.* Vol 28 (1): 3.

Andrews, G., French, K. and Wilkinson, C. (1999), Appropriately trained nurses are competent at inserting intrauterine devices: an audit of clinical practice, *European Journal of Contraception and Reproductive Health Care.* Vol 14 (1): 41–44.

Armstrong, N. and Donaldson, C. (2005), *The Economics of Sexual Health.* London: fpa.

Dawe, F. and Rainsbury, P. (2003), Contraception and Sexual Health. HSM. London.

Dennis, J. and Hampton, N. (2002), IUDs: Which device? *Journal of Family Planning and Reproductive Health Care.* Vol 28 (2): 1–9.

Department of Health (DH). Judicial Review of Emergency Contraception. *R v Secretary of State for Health* (defendant) & Schering Health Care Ltd (2) Family Planning Association (interested parties), Ex Parte John Smeaton (on behalf of The Society for the Protection of Unborn Children) (claimant) (2002) CrimLR665 at http://www.dh.gov.PolicyAndGuidance/healthAndSocialCar eTopics?sexuaHealthgeneralInformation?sexualhealthgeneralArti cle?fe/en

Edwin, B. (2006), Condoms for HIV prevention do not lead to earlier sex, more sex, or more partners, meta-analysis concludes. Available at www.aidsmap.com/en/news/

Faculty of Family Planning and Reproductive Health Care (FFPRHC) (2000), Guidance – The copper intrauterine device as long-term contraception, *Journal of Family Planning and Reproductive Health Care.* Vol 30 (1): 29–42.

Faculty of Family Planning and Reproductive Health Care (FFPRHC) Clinical Effectiveness Unit. New Product Review (April 2003), Desogestrel-only pill (Cerazette) at www.ffprhc.org.uk

Faculty of Family Planning and Reproductive Health Care Clinical Effectiveness Unit (FFPRHC) (2004), Contraceptive choices for young people. *The Journal of Family Planning and Reproductive Health Care.* Vol 30 (4): 237.

Faculty of Family Planning and Reproductive Health Care Clinical Effectiveness Unit (2006), FFPRHC Guidance: Emergency contraception (April 2006), *Journal of Family Planning and Reproductive Health Care*. Vol 32 (2): 121.

Faculty of Family Planning and Reproductive Health Care (FFPRHC) Clinical Effectiveness Unit (2006), Emergency contraception, *Journal of Family Planning and Reproductive Health Care*. Vol 32 (2): 121 and www.ffprhc.org.uk/publications

Faculty of Family Planning and Reproductive Health Care (FFPRHC) (2007), Male and Female Condoms. Clinical Effective Unit. www.fsrh.org

fpa (2003), The contraceptive patch at http://fpa.org.uk/guide/contraceptive/patch cited 06.01.3

fpa (2007) leaflet – your guide to sterilisation. www.fpa.org.uk

fpa leaflet – your guide to the contraceptive patch.

fpa leaflet – your guide to the progestogen-only pill. Available at www.fpa.org.uk

Guillebaud, J. (2001), *Contraception: Your Questions Answered*. London: Churchill Livingston, p. 97, 102.

Hannaford, P. *et al*. (2007), Cancer risk among users of oral contraceptives: cohort data from the Royal College of General Practitioner's oral contraception study. *British Medical Journal*. www.bmj.org.uk

Herring, R. (2003), *Talking Cock: A Celebration of Man and His Manhood*. London: Edury Press.

Hills, S.D., Marchbanks, P.A., Tylor, L.R. and Peterson, H.B. (1999), Post-sterilization regret: findings from the United States Collaborative Review of Sterilization, *Obstetrics Gynecology*. Vol 93: 889–895.

Lande, R.F. (1995), New are injectables. Population Reports. Series K, No. 5 Baltimore MD John Hopkins School of Public Health, Population Information Program, August 1995: 1–31 cited in the *Journal of Family Planning and Reproductive Health Care* (2002), Vol 28 (1): 7–11.

McGuire, A. and Hughes, D. (1985), The economics of family planning services. Family Planning Association. London.

Population Action (2002), http://www.populationaction.org

Rosindell, A. (2005), Questions asked by Andrew Rosindell MP to the Secretary of State for Health. What the total cost of NHS funded abortions was in each year since 1997. Question answered on 23 November 2005 in the House of Commons.

Royal College of Nursing (2007), Inserting and removing subdermal contraceptive implants. Available at www.rcn.org.uk/publications or RCNDirect on0845 772 6100 code 002 240

Trussell, J. and Guthrie, K. (2007), Talking straight about emergency contraception, *Journal of Family Planning and Reproductive Health Care*. Vol 33 (3): 139.

United Nations Population Fund (UNFPA), Web site State of the World population. Available at www.unfpa.org/swp/2005/english/ch1/index.htm cited in Jacobstein, R. (2007), Long-acting and permanent contraception: an international development, service delivery perspective, *Journal of Midwifery & Woman's Health*. Vol 52 (4): 361.

Woolf, A.D. (1998), *Osteoporosis: A Clinical Guide*, 2nd Edition, London: Martin Dunitz, p. 45 cited in the *Journal of Family Planning and Reproductive Health Care* (2002) Vol 28 (1): 7–11.

FURTHER READING

Affanti, B. (2002), Injectable contraceptives: a worldwide perspective, *Journal of Family Planning and Reproductive Health Care*. Vol 28 (1): 3.

Agrawal, A. and Robinson, C. (2003), Spontaneous snapping of an Implanon® in two halves *in situ*, *Journal of Family Planning and Reproductive Health Care*. Vol 29 (4): 238.

Asker, C. *et al.* (2006), What is it about intrauterine devices that women find unacceptable? Factors that make women non-users: a qualitative study. *Journal of Family Planning and Reproductive Health Care*. Vol 32 (2): 89.

Audet, M., Moreau, W.D. *et al.* (2001), Evaluation on contraceptive efficacy and cycle control of a trans-dermal contraceptive patch vs an oral contraceptive, *Journal of the American Medical Association*. Vol 258 (18): 2347–2354.

Bacon, L. *et al.* (2003), Training and supporting pharmacist to supply progestogen-only emergency contraception, *Journal of Family Planning and Reproductive Health Care*. Vol 29 (2): 17.

Bannister, L. *et al.* (2007), Is the Faculty of Family Planning and Reproductive Health Care Guidance on emergency contraception being followed in general practice? An audit in the West Midlands. *Journal of Family Planning and Reproductive Health Care*. Vol 33 (13): 195.

Bounds, W. *et al.* (2002), Observational series on women using the contraceptive Mirena® concurrently with anti-epileptic and other enzyme-inducing drugs, *Journal of Family Planning and Reproductive Health Care*. Vol 28 (2): 79.

Bragg, T. *et al.* (2006), Implantable contraceptive devices: *primum non nocere*, *Journal of Family Planning and Reproductive Health Care*. Vol 32 (3): 190.

Cox, M. (2002), The difficulties of intrauterine contraceptive research, *Journal of Family Planning and Reproductive Health Care*. Vol 28 (2): 55.

Cox, M. *et al.*, (2002), Clinical performance of the Nova T380® intrauterine device in routine use by the UK Family Planning and Reproductive Health Research network: 5-year report, *Journal of Family Planning and Reproductive Health Care*. Vol 28 (2): 69.

Department of Health (DH) (2004), Best practice. Guidance for doctors and other health professionals in the provision of advice and treatment to young people under 16 on contraception, sexual and reproductive health. Available at www.gov.uk/publication

D'Souza, R. *et al.* (2003), Comparative controlled trail assessing the acceptability of GyneFix® versus Gyne-T 3805® for emergency contraception, *Journal of Family Planning and Reproductive Health Care*. Vol 29 (2): 23–29.

Edouard, L. (2004), Progestogens: the good, the bad and the ugly, *Journal of Family Planning and Reproductive Health Care*. Vol 30 (4): 268.

Eskandar, S. and Eckford, S.D. (2003), Intravesical migration of a GyneFix® intrauterine device, *Journal of Family Planning and Reproductive Health Care*. Vol 29 (4): 237.

Faculty of Family Planning and Reproductive Health Care (FFPRHC) (2004), Contraceptive choices for young people, *Journal of Family Planning and Reproductive Health Care*. Vol 30 (4): p. 237.

Farmer, M. and Webb, A. (2003), Intrauterine device insertion-related complications: Can they be predicted? *Journal of Family Planning and Reproductive Health Care*. Vol 29 (4): 227.

fpa leaflet – your guide to contraceptive injections from www.fpa.org.uk

fpa leaflet – your guide to diaphragms and caps.

fpa leaflet – your guide to the contraceptive implant.

fpa leaflet – your guide to the IUD.

fpa leaflet – your guide to the combined pill. Available at www.fpa.org.uk

Fraser, I. (2006), The challenges of location and removal of Implanon® contraceptive implants, *Journal of Family Planning and Reproductive Health Care*. Vol 32 (3): 151.

Gbolade, B. (2002), Depo-Provera and bone density, *Journal of Family Planning and Reproductive Health Care*. Vol 28 (1): 7.

Guillebaud, J. (2001a), *Contraception: Your Questions Answered*, 3rd Edition, London: Churchill Livingstone, p. 102.

Guillebaud, J. (2001b), *Contraception: Your Questions Answered*. London: Churchill Livingstone, p. 97.

Harrison-Woolrych, M. and Woollet, J. (2003), Progestogen-only emergency contraception and ectopic pregnancy, *Journal of Family Planning and Reproductive Health Care.* Vol 29 (1): 5.

Ho, P.C. and Kwan, M.S.W. (1993), A prospective randomized comparison of levonorgestrel with the Yuzpe regime in post-coital contraception, *Human Reproduction.* Vol 8 (3): 389.

Ikomi, A. *et al.* (2002), Efficacy of the levonorgestrel intrauterine system in treating menorrhagia: actualities and ambiguities, *Journal of Family Planning and Reproductive Health Care.* Vol 28 (2): 99.

Ismail, H., Mansour, D. and Singh, M. (2006), Migration of Implanon®, *Journal of Family Planning and Reproductive Health Care.* Vol 32 (3): 157.

Konamme, S. *et al.* (2006), A novel device for removal of the retained intrauterine device, *Journal of Family Planning and Reproductive Health Care.* Vol 32 (2): 87.

Lee, D. (2007), Training to fit intrauterine devices/intrauterine systems for general practitioners: Is there an alternative method of service delivery? *Journal of Family Planning and Reproductive Health Care.* Vol 33 (3): 205.

Lloyd, K. and Gale, E. (2005), Provision of emergency hormonal contraception through community pharmacists in a rural area, *Journal of Family Planning and Reproductive Health Care.* Vol 31 (4): 297.

MacGregor, A. *et al.*, (2002), Prevention of migraine in the pill-free interval of combined oral contraceptives: a double-blind, placebo-controlled pilot study using natural oestrogen supplements, *Journal of Family Planning and Reproductive Health Care.* Vol 28 (1): 27.

Mavranezouli, I. and Wilkinson, C. (2006), Long-acting reversible contraceptives: not only effective, but also a cost-effective option for the National Health Service, *Journal of Family Planning and Reproductive Health Care.* Vol 32 (1): 3–4.

National Institute for Health and Clinical Excellence (NICE) (2005), The effective and appropriate use of long acting reversible contraception. Available at www.nice.org.uk/pdf/CG30

Novikova, N., Weisberg, E., Stanczyk, F.Z. and Croxto, H.B. (2007), *Contraception.* Vol 75 (2): 112–118.

Nursing and Midwifery Council (2007), Medicines Management at www.nmc.org.uk

Reuter, S. (2003), The emergency intrauterine device: an endangered species, *Journal of Family Planning and Reproductive Health Care.* Vol 29 (2): 5.

Rowlands, S. (2003), Newer progestogens. *Journal of Family Planning and Reproductive Health Care.* Vol 29 (1): 13.

Ryan, P.J., Singh, S.P. and Guillebaud, J. (2002), Depot medroxyprogesterone and bone mineral density, *Journal of Family Planning and Reproductive Health Care*. Vol 28 (1): 12.

Singh, M., Mansour, D. and Richardson, D. (2006), Location and removal of non-palpable Implanon® implant with the aid of ultrasound guidance, *Journal of Family Planning and Reproductive Health Care*. Vol 32 (3): 153.

Smith, L. (2006), Contraception in the 16th century, *Journal of Family Planning and Reproductive Health Care*. Vol 32 (1): 59.

Smith, J. *et al*. (2003), Cervical caner and use of hormonal contraceptives, *The Lancet*. Vol 361 (9364): 1159.

Sutherland, C. (2001), *Women's Health. A Handbook for Nurses*. London: Churchill Livingstone.

Taylor, B. (2003), The role of the pharmacist in emergency contraception, *Journal of Family Planning and Reproductive Health Care*. Vol 29 (2): 7.

The Faculty of Family Planning and Reproductive Health Care (FFPRHC) Clinical Effectiveness Unit (CEU) (2006), Emergency contraception. Available at www.ffprhc.org.uk/publications

The US based OrthEvra have some interesting commercial adverts viewable via www.contracpetiive-patch.orthevra.com/video_play.html

Tolcher, R. (2003), Intrauterine techniques: contentious or consensus opinion, *Journal of Family Planning and Reproductive Health Care*. Vol 29 (1): 21.

Walling, M. (2005), How to remove impalpable Implanon® implants, *Journal of Family Planning and Reproductive Health Care*. Vol 31 (4): 320.

USEFUL WEBSITES

www.fsrhc.org.uk
www.brook.org.uk
www.dh.gov.uk
www.fpa.org.uk
www.ffprhc.org.uk

Abortion

6

Kathy French

INTRODUCTION

This chapter will address abortion, one of the most controversial procedures in healthcare provision. The aim of this chapter is to inform the reader about the law surrounding abortion, recent statistics around abortion, available methods of abortion and follow-up care together with contraception choices afterwards.

Having read this chapter, the reader should be able to understand the current law around abortion and the rights of the pregnant woman. The reader should also be familiar with the referral pathways for abortion care and be able to signpost women to services should she decide that is the option for her.

LEARNING OUTCOMES

After reading this chapter the reader will:

❏ Understand the current law on abortion
❏ Understand the methods of abortion available to women
❏ Appreciate the ethical and moral dimensions of abortion

Abortion has always been a debated topic within society and at the heart of the debate lies the issues of competing rights, those of the pregnant woman and those of the unborn child. Some members of society believe that abortion amounts to the murder of the unborn child whilst others consider that abortion is the right of women and it is her alone who should make the decision regarding her pregnancy. Abortion is the termination of a pregnancy which may have been unplanned resulting from contraception failure or as the result of unprotected sexual intercourse. Occasionally, abortion is requested after a planned pregnancy but where the circumstances have changed dramatically for the woman, making the continuation of the pregnancy very difficult for her and her existing family.

Abortion is also available to women who discover that their unborn child is suffering from severe abnormalities. In such cases, the pregnancy may be beyond 24 weeks and this can be very distressing for all concerned. Such cases are generally cared for within the midwifery services and will not be addressed here. Women with a wanted and planned pregnancy who are having their pregnancy terminated because of foetal abnormality should not be cared for with women who are seeking an abortion because of an unintended/unplanned pregnancy.

It is estimated that some 46 million abortions take place worldwide each year and at least 40% occur in unsafe circumstances leading to a high risk of maternal mortality and morbidity accounting to 68,000 deaths (IPPF, 2006)

In England, Scotland and Wales, it is not a matter whether abortion should be allowed or not as the practice of abortion (legally) has been with us since the passing of the Abortion Act in 1967. The evolution of the abortion legislation to decriminalise abortion lies in the Offences Against the Person Act 1861, sections 58 and 59 which proscribes procuring the miscarriage of a woman by a third party. The Act makes no distinction between criminal and therapeutic activity and has not been repealed. The next break in the law came almost 70 years later with the passing of the Infant Life (Preservation) Act in 1929 which introduced the offence of child destruction or causing the death of a child capable of being born alive. The next major mention of abortion came with the *R v Bourne* case in 1939. This case related to Dr Bourne who performed an abortion on a 15-year-old girl who was pregnant as a result of a malicious rape. Whilst Dr Bourne was indicated under the Offences Against the Person Act of 1861, the judge linked this Act and the Infant Life Preservation Act 1929 and ruled that in a case brought under the 1861 Act, the burden rested on the Crown to satisfy the jury that the defendant did not procure the miscarriage on the girl in good faith for the only purpose of preserving her life (Mason and McCall-Smith, 1999). Dr Bourne was acquitted, recognising that the woman's life included her mental health as well as her physical health. From that time, abortion was performed quietly by doctors willing to help women, many of whom paid for the procedure. Women without funds resorted to the help of other 'experts' in the field. These were often referred to as backstreet abortions, see film Vera Drake for a greater understanding of the time before the Abortion Act 1967.

Prior to the Abortion Act in 1967, it is estimated that between 100,000 and 150,000 illegal or 'backstreet' abortions took place each year in the United Kingdom resulting in around 40 deaths a year and many more injuries (Education for Choice, 2007). It was because of the high rates of maternal deaths and complications of abortion that the Abortion Act came into being.

The Abortion Act 1967 has been significantly amended by the Human Fertilisation and Embryology Act 1990, section 37 states that a person shall not be guilty of an offence of abortion and that legal termination of pregnancy may be carried out, provided that two registered medical practitioners agree that:

(1) **Up to 24 weeks**
   - The continuance of the pregnancy would involve risk, greater than if the pregnancy were terminated, of injury to the physical or mental health of the pregnant woman or any existing children of her family. (The woman's actual or reasonably foreseeable future environment may be taken into account.)

(2) **With no limits**
   - The termination is necessary to prevent grave permanent injury to the physical or mental health of the pregnant woman.
   - There is a risk to the life of the pregnant woman, greater than if the pregnancy were terminated.
   - There is substantial risk that if the child were born it would suffer from such physical or mental abnormalities as to be seriously handicapped.

The law also requires that abortion takes place on NHS or approved premises, for example in a private abortion clinic.

It must be remembered that this law does not extend to Northern Ireland (NI), the law relating to abortion in NI is contained in sections 58 and 59 of the Offences Against the Person's Act 1861 and in section 25 (1) of the Criminal Justice Act (NI). Abortion is performed in NI but only in exceptional circumstances, for example, if the life or the mental or physical health of the woman is at serious risk or grave risk and if there is an actual risk that the baby will be severely handicapped. For further exploration of the law in NI around abortion, the Department of Health, Social Services and Public Safety published draft guidelines and best medical practice for those healthcare professionals and others faced with women seeking advice on abortion. The existing Abortion Act works reasonably well in England, Wales and Scotland in comparison to other Western European countries where the law appears more liberal. In some countries, abortion is more or less available on demand up to 12 weeks but more difficult for women with later gestations.

There have been some attempts in the House of Commons to reduce the upper limit of 24 weeks for abortion to 20 weeks and for women to have a 'cooling-off' period to consider their options. These motions have been rejected but with more and more visual images of the developing foetus and better technology for sustaining life, these demands may continue. In May 2008, attempts to reduce the upper limit of 24 weeks to either 12, 16, 18, 20 or 22 weeks was voted against by the MPs.

In March 2007, there was a motion to force doctors offering abortion or contraception to under 16 year olds to inform the parents, but this was rejected with a majority vote to retain the current guidelines guaranteeing confidential advice to young people. The DH document titled *Best Practice Guidance for Doctors and other health professionals on the provision of Advice and Treatment to Young People under Sixteen on Contraception, Sexual and Reproductive Health* at www.doh.gov.uk (DH, 2004) is aimed at helping those providing treatment to young people. More recently, the British Medical Association (BMA) in June 2007 passed a motion at their Annual Representative Meeting in favour of:

> That this meeting calls for legislation to be amended so that first trimester abortion would be available on the same basis of informed consent as other treatment and therefore without the

need for two doctor's signatures and that changes in relation to first trimester abortion should be not adversely impact upon the availability of later abortion (BMA, 2007).

This meeting, however, rejected the proposal that nurses and midwives should carry out abortions.

Abortion is one of the most regulated medical procedures requiring the agreement of two registered medical practitioners acting in 'good faith' on behalf of the woman, to sign the legal paperwork.

Abortion, as stated earlier, is part of the wider sexual health care and services and is included in the recommended standards for sexual health from the Medical Foundation for acquired immunodeficiency syndrome and Sexual Health. These standards recommend that women should be able to access abortion ideally within 2 weeks, but within a maximum of 3 weeks, of initial contact with healthcare providers (MedFash, 2005). Abortion provision should be Human Rights compliant and the same standard of provision and care should be available to women regardless of postcode.

In 2004, the Royal College of Obstetricians and Gynaecologists published an evidenced-based clinical guideline titled, The Care of Women Requesting Induced Abortion. The key aim of the guideline is to ensure that all women considering induced abortion have access to a service of uniformly high quality and that the guideline be implemented across all relevant healthcare sectors and to promote a consistent standard, regardless of the sectors in which an individual woman is managed (RCOG, 2004).

Some women may seek late abortions for a variety of reason, for example, the very young pregnant woman; women in denial, stigma, fear, change in the relationship or circumstances; women with medical conditions where abortion may exacerbate the condition and women who have had a diagnosis of foetal abnormalities. Another reason for delayed abortion may rest with inadequate service provision and/or poor referral systems where women are directed to the wrong service and thereby time wasting.

The Department of Health (2008) published an evaluation of early medical abortion (EMA) which was piloted in two sites. This report is available at www.dh@prolog.uk.com.

COUNSELLING/SUPPORT

Women considering abortion should have access to supportive, empathetic counselling provided by staff trained in the speciality and should include discussion around all the options available. The counselling should respect the religious and cultural needs of the woman concerned and their partner. Some women may need additional help and support, especially those women who may be under pressure from partner, family or other members of society or those who may be suffering from a medical condition.

During the sessions the woman should be informed about the process and procedures involved, this may depend on the gestation, pre-procedure blood tests and screening, medications used, ultrasound scanning, length of stay in the hospital/clinic, contraception for the future and most importantly any complications during, immediately or later following the procedure. Discussion on alternatives to abortion should also be discussed, as some women may want permission to continue with the pregnancy. Following counselling, some women may want to think about the options for a few days before proceeding with the abortion and this should be respected. It may come to light that the pregnancy is the result of sexual abuse or there is suspicion of abuse and onward referral may be necessary. It is important to remember that the majority of women are in consensual relationships; however, there may be some who have been the victim of sexual abuse or violence, especially the younger woman or indeed the older vulnerable woman. Those healthcare professionals involved in the counselling process should be especially trained in child protection issues, take appropriate action and follow their local and national policies on child protection matters. All staff working with young people should have training in child protection and be familiar with the referral process for their area.

REFERRAL

If a woman suspects she is pregnant, it is important that she has the pregnancy confirmed and if in doubt then pregnancy tests can be performed at any sexual health/contraception clinic or in most general practices and referral should be made as soon as possible. Some women will purchase a pregnancy test from the pharmacists believing she may be pregnant. Women should not be delayed in seeking advice and help at the earliest opportunity in order that they may have the abortion as soon as possible. Whilst early abortion is a safe procedure when performed by a skilled practitioner, but the sooner it is performed the better as the risk of complications increase with increasing gestation. Women, however, should not be pressurised if unsure. Every effort should be made to ensure all women know this and they can act sooner rather than later. The younger the individual the more likely they may delay seeking help and some young women may live in hope that their period will return and they can be in denial or be fearful about being pregnant. Healthcare professionals should be aware of the referral process in their area in order to get women referred as soon as possible. Some areas have contracts with private providers, for example, Marie Stopes International (MSI) or the British Pregnancy Advisory Services (BPAS). Some women may be pressurised to continue with the pregnancy whilst others may be pressurised to seek abortion and they should be seen on their own and given the opportunity to express what they want without coercion. Others may not have a good command of the language and will need the services of an interpreter (non-family) to help them fully understand the options, procedures and any complications before they can make an informed choice.

CONSENT FOR ABORTION

The issue of consent to abortion is the same as consenting to any other medical procedure but women will need to have all the information in order to make a decision. For consent to be valid in law, the person must be competent to make the decision, have enough information to make the decision and be free from coercion. Healthcare professionals have a responsibility to ensure that they take all reasonable action to inform the woman seeking abortion about the procedure, other options, any complications, screening or tests involved and medications used. Women are often concerned about future fertility following abortion and this will need to be addressed.

Young women under the age of 16 years of age may seek an abortion without parental knowledge or/and consent. Every effort should be made to encourage the young woman to involve the parent/carer. The younger the person the more important this partnership should be. Should a young person for whatever reason, following counselling decide not to involve the parent, then the assessment of Gillick competence will apply. Guidelines following the well-published Gillick case in 1985 related to the provision of contraception and these are known as the Fraser guidelines stated by Lord Fraser after the Gillick case. A greater exploration of Gillick and the mature minor will be addressed in greater detail in the consent and confidentiality chapter. Following the Gillick case, the House of Lords issued guidance via the Department of Health and Social Security in the form of a Health Circular (HC(FP) (86)1) which outlined the position of the mature minor and stated that:

> any competent young person, regardless of age can give valid consent to medical treatment.

Whether the young person is mature enough to proceed without parental knowledge and consent would be a matter of individual assessment following counselling with the young woman involved, however, it would be unlikely that a young woman would go ahead with abortion without the support of her parent/carer. The counsellor would explore the reasons why the parent should not be involved, these may be religious or cultural reasons and if it was felt that proceeding without the consent of the parent was in the 'best interests' of that individual young woman, the lead consultant would decide the way forward on each individual case. Women regardless of age, do not legally need the consent of their partner to have an abortion.

Healthcare professionals have an obligation to encourage any young person to involve her parents or carers but should not go against the wishes of the young person but respect their autonomy. These can be competing tensions, the right of the young person and the support of the parent, and not all young people live in supporting families but the majority do and most parents would want to support their young people at this difficult time.

The legal age of consent in England, Wales and Scotland is 16 years and in NI it is 17 years.

CONFIDENTIALITY

The right to confidentiality will apply to abortion and every effort should be made to ensure the woman's confidence is not breached. In terms of the mature minor, if the young woman is capable of giving consent to the procedure using Gillick Competence under the Fraser guidelines, she is also entitled to confidentiality. The most recent case law relating to the mature minor and abortion was in 1986 (Judge-Butler-Sloss, 1986). A 15-year-old girl wanted to have an abortion against her parent's wishes and Judge Butler-Sloss ruled that she was mature enough to seek advice and information and that being the case, she was also entitled to confidentiality stating that:

> I am satisfied she wants this abortion; she understands the impli-
> cations of it (Judge-Butler-Sloss, 1986).

That said, it is important that issues of sexual abuse or suspected sexual exploitation is addressed. Child protection training and clear protocols must be in place for healthcare professionals in order that they can take the appropriate action if needed and know how to refer onwards. It is difficult to state precisely how a woman may present to a health professional if she is being abused therefore it is with experience and training that teams will be able to make an assessment during the counselling process. The young woman may attend with an older man who is very controlling and ensures she does not have a voice for herself. She may appear withdrawn, non-communicative and be frightened about what may happen. Every possible effort must be made to ensure that these issues are addressed.

The majority of young women will be able to account for the pregnancy in terms of their partner and may be accompanied and supported. Others may be very vague and find it difficult to talk about that aspect of the situation. A young girl will not on the whole confide if she is being abused sexually as she may be threatened by the abuser, should she share this information with a third party. In all these situations, it is important to see the young woman on her own to ensure that the decision to terminate the pregnancy is hers and hers alone, a caring parent may think it more appropriate for an abortion whilst the young woman may want to continue with the pregnancy. Whatever decisions she makes this should be supported, whether to continue the pregnancy or choose an abortion, neither will be an easy decision but they must be hers alone. Generally, healthcare professionals will not have to deal with these difficult matters often but from time to time, they will arise and staff will need appropriate training and the skills to ensure the process does not do greater harm to the woman concerned by inappropriate referral. The key concern throughout the process is for the well-being of the young woman.

CASE STUDY 1

A young girl attended the abortion clinic aged 13 years; she was 7–8 weeks pregnant. Her father accompanied her and was able to tell the staff that she missed a period. He knew this as he bought her sanitary protection and performed the pregnancy test at home.

The father did most of the talking and advanced answers to any questions asked. It was important to see the young girl alone. It would appear from the story that this young girl had a 'one episode' of sex with a young man who she did not know. They both refused to have any referral to social services in line with the local protocol but this was done with their knowledge but without their consent. Following the abortion, the products of conception were retained for forensic examination and DNA profiling. The case went to court some time later and on DNA evidence, the father was convicted.

Whilst the father in this case was in a supporting role, it was felt that part of his behaviour was inappropriate in dealing with his daughter and it was the skill of the counsellor that lead to a referral being made to social services.

These cases are not common but a 13-year-old pregnant girl presenting with a vague story of how she conceived raised questions for the counsellor. Most young girls are accompanied by a parent or a boyfriend and are able to articulate how the pregnancy happened, whether lack of contraception or failed contraception.

These two cases differ greatly, the first young woman was young and her story did not add up whilst the second young woman was clear about what happened and was supported by both mother and partner. The majority of people attending

---

CASE STUDY 2

A 15-year-old student came to clinic with her mother and regular boy-friend. The scan confirmed that she was 7 weeks and 3 days preg-nant. She and her boyfriend had been together for 1 year. The mother said she would support whatever decision they made. The young girl was seen alone and she was sure she did not want to continue with the pregnancy. She said she did not want her mother to be respon-sible for caring for the child whilst she finished her studies and then went to university. Her mother also cared for her maternal grand-mother and she felt this was unfair to her mother.

After the session, they all reluctantly agreed that abortion would be the way forward. This young girl was clear about what she wanted, she had the support of her family and there were no concerns about child protection issues.

---

services will not cause any concern but from time to time, issues of sexual exploitation or lack of consent may be suspected and every effort should be made to protect that young person. Non-consensual sexual intercourse is a key concern to those working in the field and rightly so.

Reflection time

Thinking of the presence of the father in the first case, how might you manage to see the young girl alone?

This is important otherwise you may only get one side of the story in any counselling session, be it from the mother or the father and the voice of the young person is vital.

The following strategy, whether in abortion counselling or in another area may be useful:

- Introduce yourself in the usual way
- State the purpose of the session
- Invite the parent/carer to have a say but also state something like 'before I see X on her own, is there anything you might want to say or ask?' That gives a clear message that you are keen to involve the parent/carer but must see the 'client' alone
- Suggest that the parent/carer can see you at the end of the ses-sion if they have any further questions

(*continued*)

> - You do not want to alienate the parent/carer but have them work with you for the benefit of the young person
> - Explaining that this is the protocol of your Trust/Board and the reasons behind it will help the parent/carer to understand the situation.

Generally this is all that is needed and if a parent/carer refuses to leave, you can simply say it will be difficult to move on until you see the young person alone. Most parents will accept this and bear in mind all that will be discussed by the nurse/doctor/counsellor and the young person may be shared between the young person and her parents later.

RIGHTS OF THE PROSPECTIVE FATHER
Claims that the prospective father should have an equal say in abortion decisions reflect an increased recognition of individual autonomy in all aspects of healthcare provision but what rights do prospective fathers really have in law? The English position was established in the case of Patten where it was laid down that a husband cannot by injunction prevent his wife from undergoing a lawful abortion (*Patten v British Pregnancy Advisory Services Trustees*, 1979). This decision was also upheld by the European Court of Human Rights. Much later in the case of *Kelly v Kelly* in Scotland, Mr Kelly tried to prevent his wife from having an abortion but failed and the abortion went ahead regardless of his wishes (*Kelly v Kelly*, 1997).

PRE-ABORTION MANAGEMENT
All women should be offered counselling as stated earlier, together with assessment of their haemoglobin concentration, blood group and in populations where sickle cell and thalassaemia are prevalent. Some abortion centres also offer screening for human immunodeficiency virus (HIV) and other blood-borne infections, for example, Hepatitis B and C. If HIV screening is offered, the women should give their consent to the procedure.

Ultrasound scanning should be available to access the gestation and to detect the presence of an extra-uterine pregnancy. Scanning should be done in a sensitive manner and not in an antenatal clinic where woman are attending with a planned pregnancy.

Sexually transmitted infection advice and screening are now commonplace in most abortion clinics with the aim to reduce the risk of post-procedure infection such as genital tract infection, including pelvic inflammatory disease is a recognised complication of abortion (RCOG, 2004). The following regimes are suitable prior to abortion:

- Metronidazole 1 g rectally at the time of the abortion plus
- Doxycycline 100 mg orally twice daily for 7 days, starting on the day of the abortion OR
- Metronidazole 1 g rectally at the time of the abortion plus
- Azithromcyin 1 g orally on the day of the abortion (RCOG, 2004).

METHODS OF ABORTION

The method of abortion will depend on the gestation, the skill of the clinician, the facilities and medication available and the preference of the woman.

Surgical methods

Vacuum aspiration is a surgical procedure where the contents of the uterus are evacuated through a plastic or a non-sharp curette and can be performed under a local or general anaesthesia. Electric or manual aspiration devices may be used. If surgical abortion is carried out using local anaesthesia, it is vital that adequate pain relief is given and the woman understands the procedure in advance. Abortion with a local anaesthesia is safer and should be available to women with an early pregnancy.

For gestations over 15 weeks, the practitioner may opt for a surgical method of abortion by dilation and evacuation (D&E) preceded by cervical preparation. This procedure must be performed by a skilled practitioner, who performs sufficient numbers of late abortions to maintain competence and skill (RCOG, 2004).

The recommendations for the RCOG are that misoprostol 400 µg are administered vaginally by either the woman or the clinician 3 hours before the abortion or gemeprost 1 mg vaginally 3 hours before the abortion or mifepristone 600 mg orally. Cervical preparations are beneficial before surgical abortions and should be a routine if the woman is aged under 18 years and for gestations over 10 weeks. These regimes will depend on the advice of the lead clinician.

Medical methods

EMA is subject to the law governing all abortions in Britain. A pregnancy can be terminated medically by the use of a combination of the antiprogestogen mifepristone and a prostaglandin, such as misoprostol or gemeprost. EMA can be carried out up to 9 weeks (63 days) and does not involve any surgery. Women may also have a medical abortion between 9 and 20 weeks but will need a higher dose of the pills mentioned earlier.

Women will have the same care at counselling as surgical methods but will not remain in hospital for so long. They will be prescribed mifepristone by a doctor and the woman will take the medication to start the abortion. The woman will return some 36–48 hours later for either misoprostol or gemeprost and most women will need no further intervention after that. If there is any doubt that the abortion is not complete, a scan will be performed to exclude an ongoing pregnancy.

The RCOG also issued guidance in 1996, which emphasises that legal abortion must not be allowed to result in a live birth and this also included guidance that for terminations after 21 weeks, the method chosen should ensure that the foetus is born dead (RCOG, 1996). The number of abortions between 20 and 24 weeks are about 2% of the total number of abortions and are usually for women, who have not been aware that they were pregnant, for example, those women approaching the menopause, the younger women who may be in denial about the pregnancy, a woman using a method of contraception where periods are often missed or finally a woman where her family circumstances have changed, which makes continuing the pregnancy difficult.

COMPLICATIONS OF ABORTION

Complications of abortion are rare in the hands of skilled clinicians; however, a woman must be informed about the possible risks in order that she makes a decision which is informed.

Immediate/Short term

- Perforation of the uterus (in surgical method it is moderate with 1–4 in 1000)

- Haemorrhage (1 in 1000 overall, less for early and up to 4 in 1000>20 weeks)
- Cervical trauma (moderate with 1 in 100)
- Failed abortion and continuing pregnancy (2.3 in 1000 for surgical abortion and between 1 and 14 in 1000 for medical abortion, depending on the regime used)
- Post abortion infection, including pelvic inflammatory infection (approximately 10% of cases) (RCOG, 2004).

Long term
- Possible regret.

There is no evidence to suggest that abortion increases the risk of breast cancer, ectopic pregnancy or infertility.

POST-PROCEDURE AND FOLLOW-UP CARE AND ADVICE
Women should be given a written account of what to expect following abortion and a list of where to go in the case of an emergency, usually the A&E department if out of hours or back to the clinic/GP or local contraception service. Most units provide women with access to a 24-hour helpline number if they feel worried or concerned about bleeding, pain or/and a high temperature. The availability of clinical assessment and emergency readmission is vital for women who may in the rare event need inpatient care following abortion.

CONTRACEPTION FOLLOWING ABORTION
Contraception should be discussed and if the pregnancy resulted from failed or poor contraception use, this would be an ideal time to discuss this. Some woman may not be familiar with all methods. Contraception should be made available to all women where abortion is provided including access to long acting reversible methods of contraception. Long acting-reversible methods will be covered in Chapter 5. Women choosing intrauterine contraception or a sub-dermal implant can have these fitted at the time of first and second trimester abortions. It is not advisable for woman to have a sterilisation at the time of the abortion as this is associated with regret by the women and also by higher failure rates. With reliable methods of contraception available to women, sterilisation should be delayed until later.

At the time of an abortion, discussion around emergency contraception should take place and women should be informed about where further supplies can be obtained. This may be the first opportunity the woman has had to discuss contraception with a provider and can provide an opportunity to address risks of sexually acquired infections with the woman and her partner.

ROLE OF THE NURSE

Nurses in contraception/sexual health, gynaecology, day surgery units and private abortion clinics provide the nursing care to women seeking and undergoing an abortion but currently nurses are not permitted to carry out the actual surgical procedure. This must be performed by a registered medical practitioner as stated in the Abortion Act 1967. In terms of medical abortion, nurses can supply (not prescribe) the medication and the woman in effect starts the procedure herself. Currently, there are demands for a change in the law to allow registered nurses/midwives working in the area to be able to perform early surgical abortions and to be able to prescribe for EMA (Argent, 2007). This advancement would enable easier access for women. The BMA discussed the possibility of allowing registered nurses/midwives to undertake the procedure in June 2007 but voted against it. Nurses have extended their role extensively since the passing of the Abortion Act in 1967, it could not be envisaged then how nurses have extended their practice, for example, in woman's health, nurses perform colposcopy, insert sub-dermal implants, fit intrauterine contraceptive devices and systems and many other procedures. It is a possibility that competent and specifically trained nurses in abortion procedures may be able to perform abortion in line with many other countries but a change in the law would be necessary. In the meantime, nurses and midwives must work within the legal framework of abortion.

Nurses who have a conscientious objection to abortion must inform their employer at the earliest possible opportunity but have a legal and professional responsibility to provide nursing care to the woman until alternative arrangements are made. Nurses and others may not opt out of providing nursing care to women before, during and after an abortion. The Nursing and Midwifery Council (NMC) have advices on conscientious objection (NMC, 2006). The Royal College of Nursing has a briefing sheet which lays out the role and responsibility of the nurse should they have an objection to abortion.

Many of the abortions carried out in England are performed in independent clinics for example MSI and BPAS with local Primary Care Trusts having contracts with them to provide the service. Nurses and others working in health and social care should be familiar with what is provided locally in order to assist women needing information. A module on abortion care is available from the Faculty of Sexual and Reproductive Healthcare.

CONCLUSION

This chapter addressed the legal framework for abortion, methods of abortion and the role of the nurse in abortion care. Readers of this chapter should be able to signpost women to timely advice because the later a women has an abortion the greater the risk of complications.

REFERENCES

Argent, V. and Pavey, L. (2007), Can nurses legally perform surgical induced abortions? *Journal of Family Planning and Reproductive Health Care.* Vol 33 (2): 79.

British Medical Association (BMA) (2007), Annual representative meeting policies. Available at www.bma.org.uk

Department of Health (DH) (2004), Best Practice Guidance for Doctors and Other Health Professionals on the Provision of Advice and Treatment to Young People under Sixteen on Contraception, Sexual and Reproductive Health at www.doh.gov.uk

Department of Health (2008), Evaluation of early medical abortion (EMA) pilot sites. Final report. Available at www.dh@prlog.uk.com or 08701 555 455

Education for Choice (2007), at www.efc.org.uk/abortion

International Planned Parenthood Federation (2006), International medical Advisory Panel (IMAP) Statement on safe abortion, *Medical Bulletin.* Vol 40 (3): 1.

Kelly v Kelly, 1997 SLT 896.

Mason, K. and McCall-Smith (1999), *Law and Medical Ethics*, 5th Edition, London: Butterworths, p. 114.

Nursing and Midwifery Council (NMC) (2006), Conscientious objection. A–Z advice sheet. www.nmc.org.uk document ID=1562

Offences Against the Person's Act, 1861.

Paton v British Pregnancy Advisory Services Trustees, 1979 QB 276.

R v Bourne (*1939*), 1 KB 687.

Judge-Butler-Sloss (1986), 1 FLR 272, 80 LGR 301.

Royal College of Obstetrician and Gynaecologists (RCOG) (1996), *Termination of Pregnancy for Fetal Abnormality in England, Scotland and Wales.* London: RCOG Press.

The Abortion Act, 1967.

The Infant Life Preservation Act, 1929.

The Medical Foundation for AIDS & Sexual Health (MedFash) (2005), Recommended standards for sexual health. Available at www.medfash.org.uk

The Royal College of Obstetricians and Gynaecologists (RCOG), The care of women requesting induced abortion (2004) No 7. Available at www.rcog.org.uk

FURTHER READING

Abortion Review (2007), Why not decriminalise abortion altogether? Issue 22 ISSN 02627299. Published by bpas www.bpas.org

BPAS early medical abortion – A guide for practitioners. Available at www.bpas.org

fpa leaflet – Abortion your questions answered. Available at www.fpa.org.uk/home page/values

Marie Stopes International (2005), Late abortions a research study of women undergoing abortion between 19 and 24 weeks gestation. Available at www.mariestopes.org.uk

Mawer, C. and McGovern, M. (2003), Early abortions promoting real choice for women. fpa at www.fpa.org.uk

Nursing and Midwifery Council (2008), The code. Standards of conduct, performance and ethics for nurses and midwives. Available at www.nmc.org.uk

Shamash, J. (2002), Abortion: Is it a step too far for nurses? *Nursing Times.* Vol 98 (28 July 9): 12.

Wakely, G. (2007), Legal interpretation of the Abortion Act 1967: the role of nurses in surgical induced abortion. *Journal of Family Planning and Reproductive Health Care.* Vol 33 (2): 77.

USEFUL WEBSITES

www.bpas.org.uk
www.brook.org.uk
www.doh.org.uk
www.fpa.org.uk
www.fsrhc.org.uk
www.msi.org.uk
www.rcog.org.uk

Consent and Confidentiality | 7

Kathy French

INTRODUCTION

In general, this chapter will focus on the issues of consent and confidentiality, but in particular the issues of consent and confidentiality in relation to sexual health. The implications of the Sexual Offences Act will also be addressed and how the new legislation affects practice.

Aspects of the law relating to the mature minor and the vulnerable adult will be covered and how this relates to abortion care, contraception and genitourinary medicine clinics . By the end of this chapter, the reader will have a good understanding of the law related to consent and confidentiality and be able to apply it to sexual health.

Case law will be used to demonstrate how the law is used and case scenarios will be presented to show how consent and confidentiality works in the clinical setting. It is important to understand from the onset that the majority of young people engaged in sexual activity are doing so within consenting relationships. Despite commonly held beliefs, it is important to acknowledge that not all less than 16 years old are sexually active. It is of course vital to understand that some young people and indeed older vulnerable adults may be at risk of sexual exploitation; they may not be emotionally and intellectually equipped to enable them to fully comprehend the implications of relationships they are involved with and they may not even understand that things happening to them are unlawful. These are the groups of people where healthcare professionals need to know the referral process as great harm could be done by inappropriate action and the faith in services could be lost forever. It is also important to understand that chronological age alone is not always the best indicator of capacity to understand or comprehend and therefore giving valid consent. A confidential sexual health service is vital, otherwise young people will not access help or advice and may even conceal a pregnancy or delay seeking treatment for sexually acquired infections (SAIs), and this may not be in their best interests or indeed the interest of the wider community.

LEARNING OUTCOMES
After reading this chapter, the reader should be able to:

❏ Understand the issues of consent and confidentiality generally and those related to sexual health specifically
❏ Be aware of the need to refer young people who pose concerns
❏ Know when not to refer

CONSENT
The common law has recognised the principle that everyone has a right to have their bodily integrity protected against invasion from others. It will only be in very narrowly defined circumstances when this integrity should be compromised and these will be addressed later. Consent can be implied, for example, when a patient is advised that he/she needs a blood test and offers an arm in order for the sample to be taken.

The seriousness with which the law views any invasion of physical integrity is based on the strong moral conviction that everyone has the right of self-determination with regard to his/her body (Mason and McCall-Smith, 1999).

No actual physical harm need arise as it is the affront to bodily integrity that makes the conduct actionable happen. It does not matter that the touching is aimed to 'help' the client and any touching of the patient in any medical treatment is potentially a battery. Cardozo as far back as 1914, which is still valid today, described consent thus:

> Every human being of adult years and sound mind has a right to determine what shall be done with his/her own body: and a surgeon who performs an operation without the patient's consent commits an assault.

Patients need sufficient information before they can make a decision and this should include the benefits, risks and indeed any alternatives to treatment before they can give valid consent. Consent is an ongoing process and it is important to ensure that the patient/client has consented to all aspects of the treatment offered.

Consent can be given verbally or in writing but a signature on a consent form in law does not in itself prove that the consent is valid. Consent forms are now standardised and the best person to seek consent from a patient is generally the person treating or providing the care; however, consent can be obtained on behalf of other colleagues, but the person seeking consent must be familiar with the treatment/procedure proposed and be able to address any questions asked by the patient. For consent to be valid in law, it must be:

- given without coercion;
- patient is fully informed about risks, benefits, effects and any alternatives to treatment;
- patient understands the implications of what is proposed.

It will be in very limited situations where treatment will proceed without consent and this is termed 'non-voluntary' consent; for example, if a patient was involved in an accident and was taken to an A&E department and was incapable of giving consent, it would be assumed that that person would want to be 'put right' as it were and no action would ensue against a health professional. In the case of 'involuntary consent', which is extremely rare, treatment may be deemed necessary to protect the patient; a third party or indeed the wider community and some aspects of mental health may come into play here.

No adult can give consent for another adult (over 18) in law; however, in Scotland, the Adults with Incapacity Act 2000 permits an adult to provide consent on behalf of another adult who is incapacitated. The Mental Capacity Act 2005 will be implemented in 2007 and this allows an adult, in very specific circumstances, to consent for another adult in England, Wales and Northern Ireland.

The mature minor

Adults over the age of 18 years are assumed competent to give consent to treatment and in the UK law, a person's 18th birthday draws a line between childhood and adulthood (Children Act, 1989) and therefore an 18-year old will enjoy the same autonomy as any other adult in matters of healthcare provision. The Family Law Reform Act 1969 also allows young people between the ages of 16 and 18 to a limited extent to make medical decisions independently of their parents. Those young people under 16 may consent to treatment and this will be dependent upon their level of competence. Age alone is an unreliable predictor of competence and this should be judged on a case-by-case basis. The family may express a preference for treatment in the case of another family member who does not have capacity but this should not be confused with consent.

The status of the minor between the ages of 16 and 18 is clear under section 8 of the Family Reform Act 1969 and young people between those ages can consent to treatment. The age of consent in Northern Ireland is 17 years.

Unlike adults, if a young person between the ages of 16 and 18 refuses treatment, his/her wishes can be overridden by the parent or the courts. The common law does not exclude a young person under 16 from giving consent but to be valid, the consent has to be considered in the light of the important case of *Gillick v West Norfolk and Wisbech Area Health Authority* 1984. This well-known case was related to the provision of contraception, but the points made can be taken as relating to any treatment or advice and the term 'Gillick competent' is commonly used to assess the maturity of young people in contraceptive/sexual health clinics.

The court took the view that it would be a question of fact to be decided in each case whether a child seeking advice had sufficient understanding to give consent valid in law. Young people may be able to consent to one treatment, for example, emergency contraception but not to cardiac surgery. The Gillick case was decided in the House of Lords and its authority extends to Scotland as well but Scots law has gone beyond Gillick with the enactment of the Age of Legal Capacity (Scotland) Act (1991), section 2(4) known as the 'Scottish Act'. Under the 'Scottish Act', it is the young person's 16th birthday that draws the line between childhood and adulthood, not his/her 18th birthday. The Act has provided that in certain circumstances a person under the age of 16 years will be deemed to have the capacity to consent to any surgical, medical or dental treatment or procedure with the proviso that he/she is capable of understanding the nature and consequences of the proposed treatment and procedure.

The Government published a paper titled *Working Together to Safeguard Children* which outlined how agencies should work together to protect children (DH, 1999). The document stated that:

> ....forcing or enticing a child or young person to take part in sexual activities, whether or not the child is aware of what is happening. The activities may include penetrative (e.g. rape or buggery) or non-penetrative acts. They may include non-contact activities, such as involving children in looking at pornographic material or watching sexual activities, or encouraging children to behave in sexually inappropriate ways (DH, 1999).

Healthcare professionals should be familiar with the legal framework around child protection in whichever part of Great Britain they practise as these may be very different from place to place.

Fraser guidelines

These guidelines followed the well-known Gillick case and the importance of these guidelines can be found in the speech by Lord Fraser in which he said that the doctor (whilst doctor was in the wording then, it is now a given that this refers to any healthcare professional) would be justified in proceeding with contraceptive advice without parental consent, or even knowledge, provided the physician was satisfied that certain criteria were met and these are as follows:

- The young person understands the advice and has sufficient maturity to understand what is involved.
- The doctor could not persuade the young person to inform his/her parents, nor to allow the doctor to inform them.

- The young person would be very likely to begin or continue having sexual intercourse with or without contraceptive treatment.
- Without advice or treatment, the young person's physical or mental health or both would suffer.
- It would be in the young person's 'best interests' to give such advice or treatment without parental consent.

Any decision to proceed with treatment must be made on clinical grounds alone and will depend on the severity of the procedure or therapy proposed. For example, a healthcare professional would be very unlikely to proceed with major surgery on a mature minor without the consent of the parent but may well provide emergency or ongoing contraception and indeed an abortion without consent. The majority of young people would want the support of the parent for any surgery but may want to keep their sexual health matters to themselves. Consent and abortion is addressed in Chapter 6.

The Children Act 1989 sets out a list of those persons with responsibility that can consent for minors and they are as follows:

- The child's parents if married to each other at the time of conception or birth of the child.
- The child's mother but not the father unless he has acquired parental responsibility via a court order or a parental responsibility agreement or the couple subsequently marry.
- The child's legally appointed guardian.
- A person in whose favour the court has made a residence order concerning the child.
- A local authority designated in a care order in respect of the child.
- A local authority or an authorised person who holds an emergency protection order in respect of the child.

There is widespread confusion about consent issues amongst some healthcare professionals, some still believing that the consent of a parent is needed before an less than 16-year old can have contraception and some surgeries openly say they will not see any less than 16-year old without the parent. Others believe any less than 16-year old can consent to almost anything. The Department of Health (DH) in consultation with health professionals, police, education and social services issued guidelines for doctors and other healthcare professionals in relation to advice and treatment for the under-16s (DH, 2004). These guidelines make it very clear how health professionals should act when they are approached by young people less than 16 years. Any non-consensual sexual activity is a concern and rightly so but is not the norm and most young people are in consenting relationships.

SCENARIO

A 15-year-old Eastern European woman attends the clinic; she has limited English. The man who comes with her says she needs 'some tests' as she might have a 'disease' and she is in a hurry. The nurse sees her and tries to get a sexual health history but because of the language difficulties, this proves problematic.

An interpreter is arranged for the next day and it becomes clear that this girl is very frightened and unable to give an accurate account; the nurse become suspicious of the lifestyle this woman may be involved in. It is explained to her through the interpreter that a referral to Social Services would be made and she would be linked to a specific worker. The interpreter stressed the importance of this to the young woman. The following day the nurse, interpreter and social worker met with the young woman and she admitted that she is involved in prostitution and could not escape her pimp. The team assured her that a safe house would be found for her and that she did not have to put up with that lifestyle. The police were involved and this young woman was rescued from a life of misery through the skill and experience of a nurse in the contraception clinic.

CASE STUDY

A 15-year-old schoolgirl comes to the clinic requesting for contraception; she is accompanied by her mother. She discussed her plans to use a reliable contraception method as she had been seeing her boyfriend for 10 months and knew they would soon have sex. Her mother knew the boyfriend and his family and was very fond of him. The mother wanted her daughter to do well at her GCSEs and then take A levels and proceed to university and the mother wanted to ensure her daughter did not get pregnant. The nurse had no concerns about the maturity of this young person and also she had the support of her mother.

Reflection time

These two cases differ greatly. The first case raised concerns as the young woman appeared to be pressurised by the male and she was not able to communicate very well and the nurse rightly felt concerned. By acting as an advocate for her, the nurse was able to help her escape from a life of exploitation. The second young woman was in a consenting relationship, supported by her mother and there was no need for further action.

It is important to be familiar with referring procedures and when to refer. Greater harm could be done by inappropriate referral and the trust placed in health care by young people could be destroyed. It is worth understanding that the majority of young people are involved in sexual relationships which are consensual and will not cause any concern to the professional.

CONFIDENTIALITY

Consent and confidentiality go hand in hand. Confidentiality has long been emphasised in medical and nursing practice and is still a fundamental part of care with the Royal Colleges publishing guidelines for their members. The Nursing and Midwifery Council (NMC, 2008) who regulates nursing practice states that 'you must treat information about patients and clients as confidential and use it only for the purpose for which it was given'. The NMC also mentions three occasions when a breach of confidentiality may be justified:

(1) When it is justified in the public interest (usually where a disclosure is essential to protect the patient or client of a third party from risk of significant harm)
(2) When nurses and midwives are required by law or by order of the court
(3) When there is an issue of child protection: the nurse or midwife must act at all times in accordance with national and local policies.

In terms of 'public interest' this must not be confused with an 'interested public', where the public might like to know the business of others, for example, the health of famous people. Whilst they may be interested to know, this is not their business of the public.

Patient information is generally held under legal and ethical obligations of confidentiality. Information should not be used or disclosed in a form that might identify a patient without their consent. Confidentiality should also be included within employment contracts as a specific requirement linked to disciplinary procedures.

The National Health Service (NHS) has a Confidentiality Code of Practice and NHS Caldicott Report in 1997 identified weakness in the way parts of the NHS handled confidential patient data and one of the recommendations made was the appointment of Caldicott Guardians. These are members of staff with a responsibility to ensure patient data is kept secure. Young people often worry about the possibility of service providers sharing with others the fact that they had visited a clinic and it is important that such services display confidentiality notices to inform young people that their visit will remain confidential. The twin issue of consent to treatment and the right to confidentiality go hand in hand and are paramount for young people; otherwise, they will not seek advice or help when they need it. If a young person has the capacity to consent to treatment and understands what is implicated, that young person is also entitled to the right to confidentiality. Confidentiality, however, is not absolute for anyone and if a healthcare professional suspects that a vulnerable person and in particular a young person is at risk of abuse or exploitation, that professional has a duty to protect the welfare, health and safety of the client and others who may be at risk of harm. Any decision to disclose information will depend on the potential harm to the client and others and not on the age of the client. As mentioned previously if a referral to social services/child protection lead is necessary, it is important that the healthcare professional follows the local policy for referral and acts in accordance with that policy. The Area Child Protection Committee is an organisation made up of representatives from general practice, nursing, medicine, education, National Society for the Prevention of Cruelty to Children (NSPCC), social services and the probationary services, which has been replaced by the Local Safeguarding Children' Boards. They have the responsibility to ensure that high standards of practice are maintained and child protection guidelines are followed when any case of abuse is suspected.

In January 2006, the result of Judicial Review into the provision of confidential sexual health advice and treatment to young people under the age of 16 was published. In effect, this review came about as a result of the DH guidelines to doctors and other health professionals (DH, 2004) which gave clarity to those working in the field of sexual health, but these guidelines were challenged by Sue Axon who was not opposed to the guidelines but felt that parents had a right to be informed at all times.

Without doubt, the best place in most cases for young people to get advice and support is from their parents but we also know that many parents do not discuss or have the training to help their young people in matters of sexual health. The judgement from the Judicial Review in 2006 is in line with current practice and upholds what nurses and others in sexual health have been doing since the Gillick case in 1984. The DH guidelines place great emphasis on health professionals to encourage young people to confide in their parents and stress the importance of parental support. There will be times, however, when the support is not there and the health professional will be concerned about the welfare of an individual young person and will need to breach confidentiality, but this should be done with the knowledge of that young person but may not always be with their consent.

The publication of the Sexual Offences Act in 2003 caused much confusion amongst healthcare professionals and others. The Sexual Offences Act, in fact, did not alter how we worked in sexual health and there was much misunderstanding about the wording. The Act was the first major overhaul of sexual offences legislation for more than a century, setting out a strong, clear and modern approach to this sensitive area of the law. The law puts the victim first and is designed to protect everyone from abuse and exploitation. In terms of adults, sex, consent is paramount and section 74 states that:

> A person consents if s/he agrees by choice and has had the freedom and capacity to make that choice (Sexual Offences Act 2003, section 74).

The new law covers matters of drink spiking, Internet grooming, prostitution, trafficking and sexual offences against people with mental disorders, including learning disabilities. The Act makes it a criminal offence to have sex with anyone under the age of 13 years and for healthcare professionals dealing with this age group who are sexually active, there is a presumption to refer to the child protection lead for the service. It will be the decision for the child protection lead to decide the next step. In law, one is judged by acts as well as omissions, and failing to act when a professional is concerned is a serious matter.

Cases of human immunodeficiency virus (HIV) and acquired immunodeficiency syndrome (AIDS) have given rise to a range of problems related to confidentiality. Sadly, today there still remains a lot of ignorance about how the virus is spread and some people believe they must do everything in their power to prevent them or others 'catching' it. One hears of drastic measures being taken in healthcare services when someone has a diagnosis of HIV. There are only a few recorded cases where a healthcare worker has been infected by a patient. Healthcare professionals should ensure they adhere to universal precautions when dealing with all patients. The DH has produced guidelines on what healthcare workers should do if they themselves are infected with HIV or other blood-borne infections (DH, 2003). These are available at www.doh.gov.uk

---

CASE LAW FOR INTEREST

The case relates to a planned disclosure of the HIV status of two doctors in the late 1980s when HIV was a most feared condition. In the case of X vs. Y, the names of two doctors being treated in hospital for an AIDS-related condition were improperly disclosed; the health authority sought and obtained an injunction to prevent their names being published in a newspaper. The health authority involved had not made out a case for forced disclosure of the source of the information but the Judge stated that such luck would be unlikely the second time and that prison would be the consequence if the informer repeated his/her betrayal of confidence stating that:

The public in general and patients in particular are entitled to expect hospital records to be confidential and it is not for any individual to take it upon himself or herself to breach that confidence whether induced by a journalist or otherwise (Mason and McCall-Smith, 1999).

CASE SCENARIO

A 16-year-old girl attends the contraception clinic requesting emergency contraception. After taking a sexual health history, it appears that the young girl is mature and understands the nature of the treatment proposed. Risks of SAIs and HIV were discussed with her. She was given emergency hormonal, emergency contraception and condoms. Ongoing contraception was also discussed and she opted to try the combined oral contraceptive. Two weeks later, her mother called the clinic to ask if she had attended and wanted to know why. The clinic nurse advised the mother that they could not share this information with her.

Parents have rights as well and it is important to engage with the mother about the importance health providers place in confidentiality.

Reflection time

You are in a ward setting and a young man is admitted with pneumonia; he looks very pale, thin and ill. You hear from other staff that he is having a test for 'AIDS'. You know enough about this condition from your lectures in the classroom and you know how HIV is transmitted. You are informed at report that the man has had a positive diagnosis for HIV, he is very ill and the senior nurse informs you that he must be nurses by staff wearing special 'red' aprons and gloves and you must also wear a mask. You notice a sticker on his notes which says infection risk. You are very concerned about these measures and how it might impact on this man and also how his visitors and relatives might react. You raise this issue with the senior nurse who argues that he is 'infectious' and might place the staff at risk. What might you do?

You could explain to her/to him that the risk to staff and others is extremely rare and explain the need for universal precautions.

You may want to explain the importance of treating this man with respect, dignity and not breaching his confidence by having special measures in place.

You may want to highlight the right this man has to confidentiality, how his relatives and others might be thinking if he is being treated differently?

You could raise the NMC code around confidentiality.

If not resolved, you could raise with your mentor or someone in authority.

Help others to understand the effect these measures may have on this man.

Provide useful documentation to help others understand the guidance.

The DH plans to publish a document of disclosure at some point in the future.

CONCLUSION

Having read this chapter, the reader should have a good understanding of the issues related to consent and confidentiality; they should also appreciate the importance of protecting the confidence of all their service users. Know when to seek advice from others and be able to refer appropriately to the relevant professionals.

REFERENCES

Age of Legal Capacity (Scotland) Act (1991) section 2 (4).

Children Act (1989) section 105 (1).

Department of Health (1999), *Working Together to Safeguard Children: A Guide to Inter-agency Working to Safeguard and Promote the Welfare of Children*, London: Her Majesty Stationary Office (HMSO).

Department of Health (2003), Infected healthcare workers. Available at www.dh.gov.uk

Department of Health (2004), Best practice guidelines for doctors and other health professionals on the provision of advice and treatment to young people under 16 on contraception, sexual and reproductive health. Available at www.dh.gov.uk

Family Law Reform Act (1969) section 8.

Gillick v West Norfolk and Wisbech Area Health Authority (1984) QB 581.

Mason, K. and McCall-Smith, A. (1999), *Law and Medical Ethics*, 5th Edition, London: Butterworths, p. 199.

FURTHER READING

Bastable, R. (2003), The sexually abused child, *The Practitioner.* Vol 247: 934.

Carter, P.Y.H. and Bannon, M.J. (2002), *The Role of Primary Care in the Protection of Children from Abuse and Neglect. A Position Paper from the Royal College of General Practitioners*. London: RCGP.

Cf, R (on application of Axon) v Secretary of State for Health (2006) HRLR 12.

Department of Education and Employment (2000), *Framework for the Assessment of Children in Need and Their Families*. London: HMSO.

Department for Education and Skills (DfES) (2004), *Every Child Matters: Change for Children*. London: The Stationery Office of Health.

Department of Health (2001). Reference guide to consent for examination or treatment. London: Department of Health. Available at www.dh.gov.uk/assetRoot/04/01/90/79/04019079

Department of Health (2000), *Framework for the Assessment of Children in Need and Their Families*. London: The Stationery Office.

Department of Health (2003), *What to Do if You're Worried a Child Is Being Abused*. London: Department of Health Publication.

Department of Health (2007), Patient confidentiality. Available at www.dh.gov.uk/en/Policyandguidance/Informationpolicy. Patientconfidentilaity

Department of Health. About the consent form. Available at www. dh.gov.uk/PolicyAndGuidnace/HealthAndSocialCareTopics/ Consnet

French, K (2006). The right to know, *Primary Health Care*. Vol 16 (1): 5.

General Medial Council (GMC) (2007), 0–18 years: guidance for all doctors. Available at www.gmc.org.uk

Home Office (2004), The Sexual Offences Act (2003). Adults: safer from sexual crime. Available at www.homeoffice.gov.uk/crime/ sexualoffences/legislation.act.html

Nursing and Midwifery Council (NMC) (2008), The code. Standards of conduct, performance and ethics for nurses and midwives. Available at www.nmc.org.uk/publications

Re W (a minor) (Consent to Medical Treatment) (1992) 4 All ER 177.

Rogstad, K. and King, H. (2003), Child protection issues and sexual health services in the UK. *The Journal of Family Planning and Reproductive Health Care*. Vol 29 (4): 182.

Royal College of Obstetricians and Gynaecologists (2004), Obtaining valid consent. Available at www.rcog.org

Sterrick, M. (2006), Competence in children – don't forget the Scottish dimension. *British Medical Journal*. 11th April published in Rapid Responses section.

Wheeler, R. (2006), Gillick or Fraser? A plea for consistency over competence in Children. *British Medical Journal*. Vol 332: 807.

USEFUL WEBSITES AND ADDRESSES

A project across the Metropolitan Police to investigate rape and support victims (www.met.police.uk/sapphire).

National Association for People Abused in Childhood (www.napac.org.uk). Helpline 0800 085 33 30.

Rape and Sexual Abuse Support Centre (www.rasasc.org.uk). Helpline 020 8683 3300.

Survivors UK who offer support for male victims of sexual violence or rape (www.survivorsuk.org.uk). Helpline 0845 1221201.

Victim Support (www.victimsupport.org.uk). Helpline 0845 30 30 900 4 (2).

Sexual Assault – Managing Disclosures of Abuse

8

Wendy Hallows

INTRODUCTION

Have you ever wondered...

> How should I respond when a client discloses sexual abuse/assault?

Disclosures of sexual abuse/assault, whether at the time of the abuse or years later, can be a very sensitive and potentially devastating event. Supportive responses from healthcare professionals can alleviate some of the negative effects of abuse, whereas unsupportive responses appear to exacerbate the negative effects of abuse, and possibly increase re-victimisation.

Whether you are a student nurse, newly qualified or new to the specialist arena of sexual health, all practitioners, at all levels, need to recognise that individuals who have experienced sexual abuse/assault may present at any time and require impartial, sensitive and meaningful support throughout any care, treatment or investigations, which should be conducted in privacy and with confidentiality guaranteed.

LEARNING OUTCOMES

At the end of this chapter you will have:

❑ An increased awareness on issues relating to sexual abuse
❑ An understanding of how to deal with disclosures
❑ An increased knowledge on the support required by victims of sexual abuse

WHAT IS SEXUAL ABUSE/ASSAULT?

Sexual abuse refers to harmful behaviours that use sex or sexuality as a weapon to control, intimidate or violate others. The formal definition is 'sexual abuse involves forcing or enticing a child or young person to take part in sexual activities including prostitution, whether or not the child is aware of what is happening. The activities may involve physical contact, including penetrative (e.g. rape, buggery or oral sex) or non-penetrative acts. They may include non-contact activities, such as involving children in looking at, or in the production of, pornographic material or watching sexual activities, or encouraging children to behave in sexually inappropriate ways' (Department for Education and Skills, 2006).

Sexual assault is any type of sexual act committed without the consent of one of the parties (RCN, 1995). The Law in relation to sexual assault covers any kind of intentional sexual touching of someone else without their consent, including touching any part of their body, clothed or unclothed, either with your body or with an object (Home Office, 2004). Even if the individual did not resist or fight back at the time of the attack, it is still an assault.

In recent years the subject of drug facilitated sexual assault (DFSA) has received increasing amounts of media attention and public interest. DFSA is often referred to as 'drug rape' or 'date rape' and the substances used (prescribed drugs, illegal drugs or alcohol) are referred to as 'date rape drugs' (Hindmarch *et al.*, 1999). These terms can be misleading as the DFSA is not always committed by the victims date (Beynon *et al.*, 2007). DFSA is defined as 'an incident of rape or sexual assault in which the victim's capacity to consent to sexual intercourse is impaired by the administration of a drug or alcohol by the assailant' (Association of Chief Police Officers, 2006).

WHO COULD BECOME A VICTIM OF SEXUAL ABUSE/ASSAULT?

Sexual abuse/assault can affect anyone: men, women and children regardless of age, race, sexuality, class, disability and occupation. It occurs in public and private places: in homes, workplaces and schools. The impact can be substantial, affecting mental, physical and sexual health.

Prevalence rates for child sexual abuse can vary depending on the definition used, that is penetration, any sexualised physical contact or non-contact, inappropriate sexual behaviour. Researches concur that there is a considerable under-reporting, which in turn has a significant impact on the prevalence rates (Coxell *et al.*, 1999). However, the research indicates that child sexual abuse is relatively common. Estimates from the literature indicate that between 7% and 30% of girls and between 3% and 13% of boys may be affected (Finkelhor, 1994; Bolen *et al.*, 1999). In studies which include non-contact abuse, high rates are reported (Meadows, 1989; Halperin *et al.*, 1996).

Furthermore, some individuals sexually abused as children can be vulnerable to re-victimisation and can find themselves in violent or abusive situations and relationships subsequently (Department of Health, 2003).

Extensive studies on rape and sexual assaults are rare and definitions for inclusion vary. The research that does exist demonstrates that, in developed countries, between 14% and 40% of females have experienced sexual violence and in the majority of cases the perpetrator is known to the victim (Department of Health, 2002). The 2000 British Crime Survey established the extent of sexual victimisation of females since the age of 16, identifying that approximately 1 in 10 females have experienced some form of sexual victimisation, including rape, and in the region of three quarters of a million females have been raped on at least one occasion (it also highlighted that these figures are probably underestimated). It identified that 'strangers' are responsible for only 8% of rapes (Myhill *et al.*, 2002). In relation to DFSA, there is little statistical information available regarding incidents, which may in part be related to under-reporting due to the side effects of some drugs (including alcohol) which may cause amnesia, resulting in the victim having little memory about the assault and being reticent to contact the police (Beynon *et al.*, 2007).

Domestic abuse accounts for 25% of all violent crimes, two out of five murders of females in England and Wales are by partners/ex-partners and approximately 30% of domestic abuse begins during pregnancy or after childbirth; existing violence often escalates at this time (Department of Health, 2003).

THE IMPORTANCE OF ASSESSMENT

Assessments of clients' needs take place in all areas of health care. However, generally clinicians only ask clients about abuse histories if they have some reason to suspect abuse. Research highlights the discrepancy between the alarming numbers of individuals who are physically and sexually abused and the relative lack of attention that is given to these topics (Carmen *et al.*, 1984).

The level of awareness about the nature and extent of sexual abuse appears low amongst professionals; individuals are rarely asked about such histories (Jacobson *et al.*, 1987; Rose *et al.*, 1991) and as a result may not receive the care and support they require. Adult survivors of abuse who have been asked about their feelings with respect to disclosure say they want to be asked/wished they had been asked (Hagan *et al.*, 1998; Richardson *et al.*, 2002).

By not initiating exploration of abuse professionals may:

- confirm an individual's belief in the need to deny the reality of their experiences;
- leave unexplored a significant factor affecting the individual's mental health, thus compromising their capacity for recovery;
- unwittingly engage in a process of re-traumatisation[1].

There are of course many reasons why professionals may not address the issue of abuse, not least that they may have been subject to abuse themselves or do not know what to do if it is disclosed (Department of Health, 2002).

To remedy this, professionals need to be able to identify individuals with abuse histories so that this can be taken into account in their care and treatment. Raising these issues routinely in assessments and subsequent care planning requires great sensitivity and understanding, together with the availability of appropriate support. Therefore professionals need the skills in how to conduct this appropriately before routine exploration is introduced. If managed in the right way, the experience of being asked and listened to can help the adult survivor; if managed incorrectly, the experience may be distressing and damaging to the survivor and result in re-traumatisation (Department of Health, 2003).

HOW TO DEAL WITH A DISCLOSURE

Due to increased media awareness of sexual abuse, individuals are gaining courage to disclose their past abusive experiences.

Individuals who are able to disclose their abuse are usually very fragile. This will be the beginning of their journey to becoming a survivor, requiring great sensitivity with the space to work through at their own pace, controlling each stage of the process.

Things to consider:

- The individual disclosing trusts you and feels that they can confide in you.
- Remember that the individual disclosing was betrayed and controlled.
- Victims are never to blame for sexual violence.

Managing a disclosure

Disclosures of sexual abuse/assault, whether at the time or years later, can be a very sensitive and potentially devastating experience. Every individual responds in a different way to abuse/assault; however, there are certain feelings that they will have in common, which can include fear, distress, anger, confusion, humiliation, numbness and guilt. The individual's feelings can vary from week to week, day to day or even minute to minute; therefore as practitioners it is essential to enable the individual to experience their feelings without fear of having them invalidated or dismissed.

The following are some tips on 'Do's' and 'Don'ts' to assist practitioners in supporting an individual at this very sensitive time of disclosure.

Do's:

- Facilitate/allow the disclosure – allow them to express, in their own words and at their own pace, what has happened to them.
- Allow the individual time, space and commitment – ensure that you give the individual your attention. Respect the individual's silences and acknowledge any anxiety, fear or anger from them. Reassure them that these feelings are normal/natural and that it is good that they are taking the opportunity to ventilate their thoughts and feelings.

- Be clear about confidentiality and inform the individual of the steps you feel you need to take to ensure their safety and well-being.
- Understand – accept and listen to what the individual is disclosing and try to understand that they were unable to prevent it from happening.
- Have empathy for the individual's feelings. Ask how they feel.
- Encourage a medical examination – whether they decide to report to the police or not, encourage a medical examination as they may require tests for SAI/HIV/pregnancy, etc.; however, remember not to put pressure on them.

Don'ts:

- Promise to keep the disclosure secret – re-enforce confidentiality, emphasising that you will only inform those who need to know. Highlighting the possible need to liaise with others in order to ensure best care and safety.
- Force or rush their disclosure.
- Look shocked at what you are being told or overwhelmed with your own feelings that the focus is now on you – get support.
- Make judgements/assumptions – they may be wrong!
- Be ignorant about sexual abuse/assault.
- Press for details/dig too deeply into the abuse – it is not our role to investigate!
- Do not touch – the individual will be feeling vulnerable following the disclosure and physical contact may result in them experiencing flashbacks.

Following a disclosure

- Follow Local Safeguarding Children Board or own organisational policies/procedures.
- Report child protection concerns as per policy.
- Document disclosure details, in as much detail as possible, using the same language as the individual used in their disclosure.
- Discuss the case with your line manager/senior colleague.
- Be aware of your own feelings, ensure that you have someone appropriate to debrief with after the disclosure and any

subsequent action – listening to the disclosure will have an impact upon your own feelings.

CONFIDENTIALITY AND CONSENT ISSUES
The Nursing and Midwifery Council (NMC) (2008), The Code. Standards of conduct, performance and ethics for nurses and midwives states that as a registered nurse, midwife or specialist community public health nurse, you must protect confidential information.

You must treat information about patients and clients as confidential and use it only for the purposes for which it was given. As it is impractical to obtain consent every time you need to share information with others, you should ensure that patients and clients understand that some information may be made available to other members of the team involved in the delivery of care. You must guard against breaches of confidentiality by protecting information from improper disclosure at all times.

You should seek patients' and clients' wishes regarding the sharing of information with their family and others. When a patient or a client is considered incapable of giving permission, you should consult relevant colleagues.

If you are required to disclose information outside the team that will have personal consequences for patients or clients, you must obtain their consent. If the patient or the client withholds consent, or if consent cannot be obtained for whatever reason, disclosures may be made only where

- they can be justified in the public interest (usually where disclosure is essential to protect the patient or client or someone else from the risk of significant harm);
- they are required by law or by order of a court.

Where there is an issue of child protection, you must act at all times in accordance with national and local policies.

CHILD PROTECTION
Any nurse, who has direct or indirect contact with children and families, has a duty to safeguard and promote the welfare of children and young people. Therefore nurses require the skills

enabling identification of children and young people at risk of possible child abuse and to act accordingly.

The NMC, the *Code of Professional Practice* (2002), states that all nurses have a duty and personal responsibility to act on best interests of a child or a young person, and to inform and alert appropriate personnel if they suspect a child is at risk or has been abused.

In 2004, the NMC published an addendum entitled Code of Professional Conduct: Standards for Conduct, Performance and Ethics, which states in section 5.4 'Where there is an issue of child protection, you must act at all times in accordance with national and local policies'. For further information and to download a copy of the publication 'What to Do if You're Worried a Child is Being Abused', visit www.everychildmatters.gov.uk or www.teachernet.gov.uk/publications (ref: 04319-2006BKT-EN).

PRE-TRIAL THERAPY

As the disclosures of sexual violence increase, so does the need for those who wish to report their abuser(s). This presents a number of concerns for those working within the legal system. The issue of pre-trial therapy has previously been viewed negatively by the criminal justice system resulting in individuals being denied therapeutic intervention by legal representatives who fear that any involvement from a therapist may prejudice the case. Practitioners have a responsibility to interact with their clients without jeopardising their chances of gaining a successful conviction of their offender. The Home Office/Crown Prosecution Service/Department of Health has produced best practice guidance of pre-trial therapy, to assist practitioners offering therapeutic intervention in these situations.

For full copy of the guidance, visit:

- For child witnesses: http://www.dh.gov.uk/assetRoot/ 04/05/94/14/04059414.pdf
- For vulnerable or intimidated adult witnesses: http://www. cps.gov.uk/publications/prosecution/pretrialadult.html

CONCLUSION

This chapter has provided knowledge and understanding of the needs of victims of sexual abuse and the importance of appropriate response to disclosures. In addition, it has provided an overview of the support mechanisms available to victims of sexual abuse and raised awareness of the impact sexual abuse may have on the lives of an individual.

SUPPORT FOR VICTIMS

- Barnardo's – 0808 100 9000 or www.barnardos.org.uk
  Barnardo's have projects nationwide. They provide services to children and young people in greatest need and influence social policy for the benefit of children.
- Burton Domestic Violence Helpline – 01283 536006
  Offering support to men and women in the Burton upon Trent area who are experiencing, or have experienced, domestic violence.
- ChildLine – 0800 11 11 or www.childline.org.uk
  ChildLine is the UK's free national helpline for children and young people in trouble or danger.
- EMERGE – 01785 225991
  Support for adult survivors of sexual abuse and their families.
- Fire in Ice – 0845 257 2645 or http://fireinice2005.co.uk/
  A self-help project run by and for the adult male survivors of childhood abuse, especially those who have suffered while in residential care. Fire in Ice aims to enable men who have suffered child abuse and their families to make positive change in their lives, also aims to make the care experience safe for children and young people.
- Kidscape – 08451 205 204 or www.kidscape.org.uk
  Committed to keeping children safe from harm or abuse. They provide practical, easy to use material for children, parents, teachers, social workers, police and community workers.
- National Association for People Abused in Childhood (NAPAC) – 0800 085 3330 or www.napac.org.uk
  NAPAC is the only national charity dedicated to helping adult survivors of childhood abuse.
- National Domestic Violence Helpline – 0808 2000 247 or www.womensaid.org.uk
  Run in partnership with Women's Aid and Refuge. To offer support, help and information to women who are experiencing, or have experienced, domestic violence.

- National Society for the Prevention of Cruelty to Children (NSPCC) – 0808 800 5000 or www.nspcc.org.uk
  NSPCC is the only children's charity in the United Kingdom with statutory powers enabling it to act to safeguard children at risk.
- Young Minds – 0800 018 2138 or www.youngminds.org.uk
  Young Minds is the national children's mental health charity committed to improving the mental health of babies, children and young people. Services include parents' information service, publications and website.
- Sexual Abuse Service, South Staffordshire Healthcare NHS Trust – 01785 257888 ext 5729
  Offers therapeutic intervention to adult survivors of sexual abuse and/or sexual assault and their families, within the South Staffordshire area. Also provides consultancy, advice, support and supervision for practitioners.
- Sexual Abuse and Rape Advice Centre (SARAC) – 01283 517185
  Support for adult survivors of sexual abuse and their families.
- Sexual Abuse and Incest Victims Emerge (SAIVE) – 01782 683133
  Support for adult survivors of sexual abuse and their families.
- Survivors UK – 0845 122 1201 or www.survivorsuk.org
  Survivors UK supports and provides resources for men who have experienced any form of sexual violence. Offers training to agencies in this field.
- Safeline – 0808 800 5005 or www.safelinewarwick.co.uk
  Safeline provides information for adults who were sexually abused as children. Also provides newsletters, forums and a helpline for survivors.
- Samaritans – 08457 909090 or www.samaritans.org
- Stop it Now! – 0808 1000 900 or www.stopitnow.org.uk
  A public information and awareness raising campaign regarding child sexual abuse. Stop it Now aims to prevent child sexual abuse by increasing public awareness and empowering people to act responsibly to protect children.

- Victim Support – 0845 30 30 900 or www.victimsupport.org
  Victim Support is the national charity which helps people
  affected by crime. They provide free and confidential support to help individuals deal with there experience, whether
  or not they report the crime.

ENDNOTE

[1] Re-traumatisation: This refers to the re-awakening and re-experiencing
of previous negative life experiences, such as child sexual abuse. This can
occur in response to a variety of stimuli or events, including those that
may be well intended. A related phenomenon is re-victimisation where
the experience of past abuse can produce the tendency for a sufferer to
develop/seek out inappropriate or further abusive situations/relation-
ships (Department of Health, 2002).

REFERENCES

Association of Chief Police Officers (2006), *Investigating Drug Facilitated Sexual Assault*. Association of Chief Police Officers. http: //www.acpo .police.uk/asp/policies/Data/Operatin%20Matisse%20report%20-%20press%20rel.%2084.doc

Beynon, C., French, K. and Delaforce, J. (2007), Alcohol is the true 'rape drug', *Nursing Standard*. Vol 21(29): 26–27.

Carmen, E., Ricker, P. and Mills, T. (1984), Victims of violence and psychiatric illness, *American Journal of Psychiatry*. Vol 141 (3): 378–383.

Coxell, A., King, M., Mezey, G. and Gordon, G. (1999), Lifetime prevalence, characteristics and associated problems of non-consensual sex in men: cross sectional survey, *British Medical Journal*. Vol 318: 846–850.

Department for Education and Skills (2006), *What to Do if You're Worried a Child is Being Abused*, London: Department for Education and Skills.

Department of Health (2002), *Women's Mental Health: Into the Mainstream*, London: Department of Health Publications.

Department of Health (2003), *Mainstreaming Gender and Women's Mental Health: Implementation Guidance*, London: Department of Health Publications.

Finkelhor, D. (1994), The international epidemiology of child sexual abuse, *Child Abuse and Neglect*. Vol 18 (5): 409–417.

Hagan, T., Donnison, J., Gregory, K., *et al.* (1998), *Breaking the Silence*, Brighton: Pavillion Publishing.

Halperin, D., Bouvier, P., Jaffe, P., Mounoud, R., *et al.* (1996), Prevalence of child sexual abuse among adolescents in Geneva: results of a cross-sectional survey, *British Medical Journal*. Vol 312: 1326–1329.

Home Office (2004), *Adults: Safer from Sexual Crime*, London: Home Office Communication Directorate.

Meadows, R. (1989), The epidemiology of child sexual abuse, *British Medical Journal*. Vol 298: 727–730.

Nursing and Midwifery Council (NMC) (2002), *Code of Professional Conduct*, London: NMC.

Nursing and Midwifery Council (NMC) (2004), *Code of Professional Conduct: Standards for Conduct, Performance and Ethics*, London: NMC.

Nursing and Midwifery Council (NMC) (2008), The Code. Standards of conduct, performance and ethics for nurses and midwives at www.nmc.org.uk

Richardson, J., Coid, J., Detruckevitch, A., *et al.* (2002), Identifying domestic violence: cross section study in primary care, *British Medical Journal*. Vol 324: 274–277.

Rose, S., Peabody, C. and Stratigeas, B. (1991), Undetected abuse among intensive care management clients, *Hospital and Community Psychiatry*. Vol 42 (5): 499–503.

Royal College of Nursing (RCN) (1995), *Responding to Rape and Sexual Assault: Guidance for Good Nursing Practice*, London: RCN.

FURTHER READING

Ainscough, C. and Toon, K. (1993), *Breaking Free*, London: Sheldon Press.

Bolen, R. and Scannapieco, M. (1999), Prevalence of child sexual abuse: a corrective analysis, *Social Service Review*. Vol 73 (3): 281–313.

Hindmarch, I. and Brinkman, R. (1999), Trends in the use of alcohol and other drugs in cases of sexual assault, *Human Psychopharmacology: Clinical and Experimental*. Vol 14: 225–231.

Home Office (2003), *Sexual Offences Act*, London: HMSO.

Home Office. URL: http://www.homeoffice.gov.uk/crime-victims/reducing-crime/sexual-offences/?version=1 [29/11/2005]

Jacobson, A. and Richardson, B. (1987), Assault experiences of 100 psychiatric patients: evidence of need for routine enquiry, *American Journal of Psychiatry*. Vol 144 (7): 908–913.

Myhill, A. and Allen, J. (2002), *Rape and Sexual Assault of Women: The Extent and Nature of the Problem*. Home Office Research Study 237 Findings from the British Crime Survey.

Stop it Now (2002), *What We All Need to Know to Protect Our Children*, Birmingham: Stop it Now UK and Ireland.

Teenage Pregnancy

9

Kathy French

INTRODUCTION

This brief chapter will focus on teenage pregnancy and provide some statistics on rates of teenage pregnancy both within the United Kingdom and other countries by a way of comparison. Some reasons will be advanced for the cause of teenage pregnancy together with government strategies and targets to reduce the rates. Mention will also be made on the benefits of school-based sex and relationship education and the role the family and wider community play in providing young people with accurate information on sexual health matters.

After reading this chapter, the reader should be able to understand some of the characteristics of teenage pregnancy, possible reasons why some people 'chose' a pregnancy during their teens and some of the mechanisms that are in place to help address it and how nurses and others might consider in their profession to help young people remain safe from sexually acquired infections (SAIs) and unintended pregnancy.

LEARNING OUTCOMES

After reading this chapter, the reader should be able to:

❏ Understand the current position regarding teenage pregnancy
❏ Understand the importance of good sex and relationship education for young people
❏ Understand the government drivers to reduce teenage pregnancy

Teenage pregnancy and parenthood is considered an important health problem both within lay and professional discourses. Over the past decade, teenage pregnancy has been regarded as an increasingly pressing 'problem' for policy makers with targets set to reduce the rates with local and national initiatives set up to address the issue.

The concept of teenage pregnancy is not new and despite the media panic and perception of teenage pregnancy as a social problem, it comes at a time when its rates in the United Kingdom are in fact declining, after peaking in the late 1960s and 1970s.

It is important to note that in some cultures getting married and having babies at a young age is the 'norm' and these pregnancies are part of the social picture. Data shows that these are often planned and wanted pregnancies and not a 'problem' for their parents.

Some aspects of the media demonise young women who have a pregnancy in their teens, believing that this is a deliberate act to gain access to housing and other benefits. There is no evidence for this assumption. Reasons for teenage pregnancies are complex and many.

There has been a shift in the sexual debut of young people towards the last century, with some choosing to express their sexuality at an earlier age. Whilst an increasing number of young teenagers are having earlier sexual intercourse, it is argued that much of this activity is associated with sexual risk taking as well, for example, non-use of condoms and/or contraception with a new or casual partner (Kane *et al.*, 2003). Early sexual activity is often regretted and if young men and women are pressurised into early sex by peers, they may not have the skills to negotiate what is best for them.

Young people's sexual activity has long been the focus of moral and policy debate and this lead to the creation of the Teenage Pregnancy Unit (TPU) in 1999. The TPU was established to implement the Social Exclusion Unit's (SEU) aims of reducing teenage conceptions. The strategy aimed to reduce conception rates among teenagers under 18 years and to ensure that young parents continue with their education or employment after childbirth (Ferriman, 1999; SEU, 1999).

Despite the creation of the TPU, teenage conception rates are much lower now than they were, for example, in the 1960s and 1970s. In 1970, the figure in England and Wales was 50 births per 1000 women and in the 1990s the rate was 30 per 1000 (Singh and Darroch, 2003). More recent figures from the TPU show a downward trend in teenage conceptions since the baseline data published in 1998. Despite the downward trend, there are parts of the country described by the TPU as 'hot spots', for example, Southwark in London. Southwark is a socially deprived part of South-East London where unemployment levels are high and opportunities limited for young people. Social exclusion has been used recently in discourses around teenage pregnancy and the term in a way has replaced poverty. Arai (2003), for example, questions the assumptions made by many researchers and policy makers, including the TPU, that reasons given for high teenage pregnancy rates are attributed to 'low expectation'. The TPU suggests that some young disadvantaged people have low expectations of education and the career opportunities and put simply see no reason not to get pregnant (SEU, 1999). Arai also questions the second and more commonly quoted assumption that poor knowledge and ignorance by young people about contraception and sexual health are the key factors to teenage conceptions. It is argued by policy makers that lack of knowledge and poor provision of contraception and abortion services is the key to reducing teenage conceptions, with little consideration as to whether pregnancy may be a chosen option for some young women. A study in Scotland in the early 1990s would suggest that there is no clear relationship between service provision and knowledge of contraception and abortion. The study explored teenage pregnancy choices in a deprived area of Scotland where pregnancy rates were six times higher than in wealthier areas and yet abortion was not the chosen option to resolve the 'problem' of pregnancy (Smith, 1993). What was interesting about this study was the fact that contraceptive services were freely available and two NHS abortion providers were located within the deprived area, suggesting that this group of teenage women had made choices for themselves about the pregnancy and not related to service provision. The rhetoric of teenage pregnancy as it emerged in the 1970s suggest that if teenagers waited until their 20s or later to have their children, they would be in a better position to provide for their children and they would be better off financially. This may be a misguided notion as disadvantaged young people may be in no way better off by waiting if the prospect of employment and inclusion does not improve. As stated earlier, there still remains a significant geographical variation in teenage pregnancy rates with higher rates in some socially deprived areas. There is evidence to suggest that young women in more affluent areas opt for abortion whereas those in areas of deprivation may choose to continue with their pregnancy.

Tony Blair, the Prime Minister in power when the TPU strategy was published, stated in the foreword that:

> 'Some of these teenagers, and some of their children, live happy and fulfilled lives. But far too many do not. Teenage mothers are less likely to finish their education, less likely to find a good job and more likely to end up both as single parents and bringing up their children in poverty. The children themselves run a much greater risk of poor health and have a much higher chance of becoming teenage mothers themselves. Our failure to tackle this problem has cost the teenagers, their children and the country dear' (SEU, 1999).

As stated earlier, reasons often given for high rates of teenage pregnancy are lack of knowledge and ignorance about contraception, including emergency contraception, lack of service provision, poor sex and relationship education and risk taking. Risk taking may be part of the lives of young people and where drugs and alcohol are also involved; the knowledge gained may not be put into practice. The Health Protection Agency (HPA) published a review of the reviews on teenage pregnancy and parenthood in 2003 and identified gaps in the evidence base in the following areas:

- Interventions aimed at specific groups, for example, people leaving care, children of teenage parents and young people from some black and minority ethnic groups.
- Interventions based in the United Kingdom.

- Needs of young men often forgotten.
- Nature of relationship between poverty, deprivation and teenage parenthood (HPA, 2003).

It is clearly evident from this publication that a lot remains unknown about the causes and the complexity of teenage pregnancy. Some young women may, in the absence of other opportunities, see no reason not to have a child at a young age when her mother and her grandmother may also have had children at a young age. There is limited evidence from the United Kingdom and the United States as to whether a teenage pregnancy is a 'problem' from the perspective of the young person. Becoming a teenage parent may for some young people be an opportunity for them to use the resources available to them and focus their attention to the future for both themselves and their baby.

Whilst there is much debate and concern about the rate of teenage pregnancy and the impression that this is a new phenomenon, it is worth remembering that throughout the 1990s teenage conception rates have been declining across the European Union with the largest decrease reported from Greece, Spain and Finland. There was an increase in the teenage pregnancy rates in the United Kingdom in 1996 and whilst it is difficult to account for that increase, there was yet another pill 'scare' in October 1995 and this may have reduced the confidence about the pill amongst some young people. The media have a responsibility to report accurately when research reaches the news.

It is often quoted that the United Kingdom has the highest rate of teenage pregnancy in Western Europe and the following table shows the declining rates in many countries, including the United Kingdom.

The Netherlands are often cited as the country with the lowest rate of teenage pregnancy but should we compare the United Kingdom with a country where a different approach to sexual health exists, the attitude is different and sex education is part of the accepted school programme and sex is discussed more openly in the Netherlands. Sex education in the Netherlands' school system is freely accepted by all. The goals and purposes of sex education are enshrined in legislation and the issues such

Country	1986	1996
Iceland	39.3	16.3
Greece	25.9	9.6
United Kingdom	23.9	22.9
Portugal	24.9	6.6
Austria	17.8	11.5
France	10.7	6.8
Norway	13.4	9.9
Ireland	12.4	2.7
Sweden	7.9	5.5
Finland	9.5	6.9
Denmark	6.7	5.7
Germany	13.0	9.6
Spain	13.1	6.1
Luxembourg	6.7	7.0
The Netherlands	5.1	4.1

Source: European Commission (2000) cited in Chambers *et al.* (2001). Courtesy of Radcliffe Medical Press.

as teenage pregnancy, SAIs and child abuse are clearly defined. This is a far cry from the way young people have access to sex in the United Kingdom; schools can refuse to allow any sex and relationship in their school, leaving young people to fend for themselves. They often gain information from inaccurate sources.

The Office of National Statistics (ONS) published the latest figures on teenage pregnancy for 2005 in early 2007 and reported that the overall rates are continuing to fall and the rates for the under-18s are at the lowest level in last 20 years (ONS, 2007). Without doubt, there is a greater awareness and availability of contraception, including emergency contraception and there is a much more effective sex and relationship education programmes in schools. The stigma for young people is reduced when sexual health is discussed in an open and frank manner.

More recently the National Institute for Health and Clinical Excellence (NICE) published a guide which focuses on one-to-one interventions to reduce the transmission of SAI including human immunodeficiency virus (HIV) infection and under 18 conceptions especially among vulnerable and at-risk groups

(NICE, 2007). Nurses and others who come into contact with young people can take a role in raising sexual health concerns with them and direct them to appropriate help and information.

SEX AND RELATIONSHIP EDUCATION

Sex and relationships education is a government backed commitment to provide sex education to young people educated in British schools, but there is, however, no consensus about what sex education should consist of in Britain (Measor *et al.*, 2000). Despite the commitment, sex education is a controversial issue with some critics arguing that providing sex and relationship education to young people at an early age will encourage them to become sexually active at an earlier age. There is, however, no research evidence to support this line and indeed the opposite is true; if young people know more, they tend to delay sexual activity and when they do become sexually active, they are more likely to use protection and to seek help. The evidence suggests that sex education can lead to a greater use of contraception and a postponement of sexual activity. The National Survey of Sexual Attitudes and Lifestyles (NASSAL) study of young people in relation to sexual health showed that the majority of young people got their information on sexual matters from school and they were less likely to report first sexual intercourse before the age of 16 (Wellings *et al.* 2000).

The aim of any programme should be to provide young people with accurate information, allow for open discussions which explore the emotional side of relationships and provide young people with skills to help them negotiate and have a positive attitude towards sexual health and well-being. As mentioned earlier, lessons can be learnt from other countries in terms of the delivery of sex and relationship education. Sweden and the Netherlands, for example, introduce sex education at an early age (Sutton, 2001). Jackson (2004) suggests that the effectiveness of sex education is dependent not on what is taught but how it is taught. Young people need to feel safe and be able to explore issues with professionals who are skilled in this area of health promotion.

School nurses are ideally placed to provide sex education within schools and there are many models of good practice;

however, there is also a shortage of school nurses in many parts of the country with one school nurse looking after several schools and this needs to be addressed.

School-based programmes which link with local services is an ideal model with young people knowing what is available locally.

Despite the positive outcomes associated with sex education within the school environment, some suggest that young men are often marginalised or forgotten, with the focus on the needs of young women. It is important to provide opportunities for young men to express their fears, hopes and aspirations in a safe place. It is often suggested that some young men do not take sex education seriously believing that they know it all anyway. This reaction may be a cover-up because young men generally do not want to be seen lacking in knowledge around sexual health. They may exhibit strong macho behaviour in the classroom but ways need to be found to help them express their concerns as well. Some evidence suggests that sex education is often directed at young women in a protective discourse, in effect with the aim of protecting them from pregnancy and SAIs. Without involving young men in discussion about their needs, the sexual health of young people will continue to be a divided landscape.

There has been much discussion in the United States on the role of abstinence in reducing teenage pregnancies and this approach has a place in sex education in terms of advising young people to delay having sexual intercourse until they are ready and not be pressurised into early sexual activity against their will or as a result of peer pressure. Many of the abstinence programmes in the United States have been driven by the moral right. Recent research from the Guttmacher Institute and Columbia University (2006) examined the role of abstinence and contraception use in the 'remarkable' decline in teenage pregnancy rates which dropped by 27% between 1991 and 2000. The research found that 86% of the decline was linked to improved use of contraception, for example, the pill and condom use, and only 14% was related to reduced sexual activity. This confirms that the direction in this country must be right, give young people the tools to make the choices and also provide accessible sexual health services for them. These services must be staffed by professionals trained to accept young people as autonomous people, to be aware of the issues of consent confidentiality and to be skilled in dealing with their changing emotional needs as they go through the often challenging transitional years.

ROLE OF THE FAMILY AND THE WIDER COMMUNITY

Everyone belongs to a family and the families are in an ideal position to help young people deal with their sexual health by talking about sexual matters in an open way and by providing them with good sexual health information. However, Rosenthal and Feldman (1999) suggest that whilst parents accept and acknowledge their responsibilities for providing guidance and education relating to sex and relationships, talking to their children about sex is difficult. Parents themselves may not have had any training or knowledge acquisition to provide help to their children and may feel embarrassed. Another major criticism of school-based sex education is that teachers are often not in control of either the subject matter or the pupils (Mages *et al.*, 2007). Sex education is not a topic like history where a teacher can simply deliver it, there are emotions, feelings, shame, guilt, embarrassment and all the religious and cultural taboos attached to it as well and training is vital.

Professionals and others working with young people can access a wide range of information about young people's sexual health by joining Brook Exchange – this is a scheme established by Brook, a health charity for young people. Members receive quarterly newsletters covering a range of topics, for example, legal issues, good practice examples and up-to-date research information. There is an annual fee which can be paid either as an individual or as part of an organisation and this offers discounted rates at Brook conferences and trainings (Brook, 2007). The fpa also provides excellent training in sexual health for professionals.

CONCLUSION

This chapter highlighted the government's approach to teenage pregnancy, provided an overview of the current sex and relationship education within schools and stressed the importance of appropriate services for young people.

REFERENCES

Arai, L. (2003a), 'Low expectations, sexual attitudes and knowledge: explaining teenage pregnancy and fertility in English communities. Insights into qualitative research,' *Sociological Review.* Vol 51 (2): 214.

Brook (2007). Available at wwwbrook.org.uk and signup@brookcentres.org.uk

Chambers, R., Wakley, G. and Chambers, S. (2001), *Tackling Teenage Pregnancy Sex, Culture and Needs*, Radcliffe Press, Oxon, p. 4.

Darroch, J.E., Singh, S. and Frost, J.J. (2003), Differences in teenage pregnancy rates amongst five developed countries: the role of sexual activity and contraception use, *Family Planning Perspectives.* Vol 33: 244–250.

Ferriman, A. (1999), England launches campaign on teenage pregnancies, *British Medical Journal.* Vol 318: 1646.

Guttmacher Institute and Columbia University (2006). U.S. Teen pregnancy rates are down primarily because teens are using contraceptives better at www.guttmacker.org

Health Protection Agency (HPA) (2003), Teenage pregnancy and parenthood: a review of reviews. Available at www.hda-online.org.uk/evidence

Jackson, P. (2004), Sexual health and young people, *Community Practitioner.* Vol 7: 48.

Kane, R. *et al.* (2003), providing information for young people in sexual health clinics: getting it right, *Journal of Family Planning and Reproductive Health Care.* Vol 29 (3): 141.

Mages, L., Salmon, D. and Orme, J. (2007), Using drama to help 'hard to reach' young people access sexual health education, *Primary Health Care.* Vol 17 (4): 41.

Measor, L., Tiffin, C. and Miller, K. (2000), *Young People's Views on Sex Education. Education, Attitudes and Behaviour.* London: Routledge Falmer.

National Institute for Health and Clinical Excellence (NICE) (2007), Oneto-one interventions to reduce the transmission of sexually transmitted infections (STIs) including HIV, and to reduce the rate of under 18 conceptions, especially among vulnerable and at risk groups. Available at www.nice.org.uk

Office of National Statistics (ONS) (2007), Teenage pregnancy rates. Available at www.ons.org.uk

Rosenthal, D. and Feldman, S. (1999), The importance of importance: Adolescents' perception of parental communications about sexuality, *Journal of adolescence.* Vol 22: 835.

Smith, T. (1993), Influences of socioeconomic factors on attaining targets for reducing teenage pregnancies, *British Medical Journal.* Vol 306: 1232.

Social Exclusion Unit (SEU) (1999), *Teenage Pregnancy*. London: HMSO.

Sutton, H. (2001), Sexual health promotion: reducing the rate of teenage pregnancy, *Paediatric Nursing*. Vol 13 (3): 33.

Wellings, K. *et al.* (2000) Sexual behaviour in Britain: early heterosexual experience. *The Lancet*. Vol 358 (9296): 1843–1850.

FURTHER READING

Baraitser, P. *et al.* (2005), Involving service users in sexual health services development, *Journal of Family Planning and Reproductive Health Care*. Vol 31 (4): 281.

Bekaert, S. (2005), Adolescents and sex. *The Handbook for Professionals Working with Young People*. Oxford: Radcliffe Publishing.

Bonell, C. (2004), Why is teenage pregnancy conceptualized as a social problem? A review of quantitative research from the USA and UK, *Culture, Health and Sexuality*. Vol 6 (3): 255.

Evans, D.T. (2000a), From 'nits' to 'crabs'. *British Journal of Nursing*. Vol 9 (18): 2022.

Evans, D.T. (2000b), Speaking of sex: the need to dispel myths and overcome fears, *British Journal of Nursing*. Vol 9 (10): 650.

French, K. (2006), The right to know, *Primary Health Care*. Vol 16: 5.

Hurst, J. (2004), Researching young people's sexuality and learning about sex: experience, need, and sex and relationship education, *Culture, Health & Sexuality*. Vol 6 (2): 115.

Tripp, J. *et al.* (2006), Sex education: the case for primary prevention and peer education, *Current Paediatrics*. Vol 16 (2): 15.

Female Genital Mutilation | **10**

Kathy French

INTRODUCTION

This chapter will address the serious matter of female genital mutilation (FGM), how it may affect the health of a woman or young girl, types of FGM performed and some reasons for the practice. After reading this chapter the reader should be aware of the practice and be able to discuss or talk to a woman about it and not show embarrassment when a woman is seeking help or when FGM is observed. Professionals should be able to direct women who need a reversal to the appropriate service for specialist help.

FGM is performed on girls between the ages of 1 week old and adolescence and has been described in the past as female circumcision. The rationale for this practice varies from setting to setting and reflects beliefs and cultural mores, including religion, health and social factors. FGM is believed to protect the virginity of the young girl, discourage female promiscuity, improve fertility, prevent stillbirth, increase a girl's chance of marriage and to maintain cleanliness (IPPF, 2001).

The precise origins of FGM are unknown but the practice of FGM dates back to 200 BC (EL Dareer, 1983); although in many parts of West Africa, the practice began in the 19th or 20th century (Duncan and Hernland, 2000). Some scholars claim it originated in the Nile valley during the Pharaonic era and dates back to 4000 years (Gilbert, 1993), cited by Marjaria (2002). Whatever the origins, this chapter aims to highlight the issues, discuss the different types of FGM, complications, the law relating to FGM and the role of the healthcare professional whenever they encounter it within the population they serve.

The World Health Organization (WHO) has classified FGM as follows:

- Type I – excision of the prepuce with or without excision of part or all of the clitoris.
- Type II – excision of the clitoris with partial or total excision of the labia minora.
- Type III – excision of part or all of the external genitalia and stitching/narrowing of the vaginal opening (infibulations).

Other procedures include pricking, piercing or incising the clitoris and/or the labia, stretching the clitoris and/or the labia, cauterisation by burning of the clitoris and surrounding tissue, scrapping of tissue surrounding the vaginal orifice (angurya cuts) or cutting of the vagina (gishiri cuts) as well as the introduction of corrosive or herbs into the vagina to cause bleeding for the purpose of tightening or narrowing it.

In Sudan, they call it *tahoor* or 'purification', in Sierra Leone, it is known as *bondo* or 'initiation'. FGM is not a rare practice but numbers are difficult to come by, but it is estimated that 130 million girls and women are thought to have undergone the procedure in more than two dozen African countries as well as parts of Asia, the Middle East and some immigrant communities in the West.

In 1994, the world's leaders met in Cairo at the International Conference on Population and Development (ICPD) and they agreed a plan to achieve 'reproductive health and rights for all' by 2015. The aim was to change the way those making the policy and delivering services thought about reproduction, rights of women and on paper much progress has been made.

The WHO estimate that worldwide the situation is as follows:

- 100 to 140 million girls and women have undergone some form of FGM, with the majority from Africa (WHO, 2000).
- An estimated 2 million or more undergo some form of FGM every year worldwide and 6000 are at risk every day (WHO, 1997).

- Many girls and women die from the short-term effects of FGM, such as haemorrhage, shock and infection.
- Many more suffer lifelong disability and may die from the long-term effects such as recurrent urinary or vaginal infections. Pain during intercourse and infertility are common consequences of FGM.

LEARNING OUTCOMES
By reading this chapter the reader should:

❏ Understand what FGM is and how this procedure is performed
❏ The negative effect this can have on a woman's health (physical and mental)
❏ The law related to FGM in the United Kingdom

COMPLICATIONS OF FGM
Complications will be listed as immediate, intermediate and long-term, and the following are cited in the Royal College of Nursing (2006) publication on FGM.

Immediate complications
- Haemorrhage, pain and shock
- Wound infection, septicaemia and tetanus
- Injury to other tissues, for example vaginal fistula
- Ulceration of genital region
- Risk of bacterial or HIV infection due to reuse of instruments without sterilisation
- Death.

Intermediate complications
- Delayed healing
- Abscesses
- Scarring/keloid formation, dysmenorrhoea and the obstruction to menstrual flow
- Pelvic infection
- Obstruction to urinary flow
- Urinary tract infection (bacteriuria is even more common than actual infection).

Long-term complications

- Psychosocial trauma and flashbacks, post-traumatic stress disorder
- Lack of trust in carers
- Vaginal closure due to scarring
- Epidermal cyst formation
- Neuromata-cut nerve endings causing permanent pain
- Pain and chronic infection from obstruction to menstrual flow
- Recurrent urinary tract infection and renal damage
- Painful intercourse (dyspareunia), lack of pleasurable sensations or orgasm and marital conflict
- Infertility from pelvic inflammatory disease and obstructed genital tract
- Risk of HIV through traumatic intercourse (where HIV is prevalent)
- Childbirth trauma-perineal tears and vaginal fistulae
- Postnatal wound infection
- Prolonged or obstructed labour from tough scarred perineum, uterine inertia or rupture, and death of infant and mother
- Vaginal fistulae as a consequence of obstructed labour.

LAW RELATING TO FGM

FGM was made illegal in Britain in 1985 with the Prohibition of Female Circumcision Act. The Act made it an offence to excise, infibulate or otherwise mutilate the whole or any part of the labia. It is also illegal under the Female Genital Mutilation Act 2003 to take a child out of the United Kingdom in order to perform FGM. The Act applies to England, Wales and Northern Ireland with Scotland passing the Prohibition of Female Genital Mutilation (Scotland) Act in 2005.

Under these Acts, it is a criminal offence to aid, abet, counsel and perform the procedure and a nurse, midwife or doctor who decided to proceed would be removed from their professional register. It is difficult to monitor FGM and prevent young girls being taken to other countries for FGM, and the Female Genital Mutilation Act (2003) states that it is no longer acceptable in the

United Kingdom even if performed in another country. The Act protects any girl who is a UK national or permanent resident from FGM anywhere in the world.

PROFESSIONAL RESPONSIBILITY

Healthcare professionals have a responsibility to ensure that they are aware of the law relating to FGM and that they provide information and support to young women and their families regarding FGM and to bring to their attention that this practice is illegal in the United Kingdom. School nurses, community health practitioners, teachers and others involved in the lives of young female children can raise this with families and if they consider a young girl or her siblings are at risk of FGM, whether having the procedure performed secretly in the United Kingdom or being 'sent' home for an 'operation', they should act to protect the young person. Child protection procedures should be in place and followed at all times. Healthcare professionals must act responsibly and with respect in such cases as families may be very offended at a reaction. Some parents may honestly believe that this procedure is the right thing to do and may not believe it contravenes the United Nations Convention on the Rights of the Child.

Whenever there is a concern that a young girl and/or her female siblings are at risk of FGM, steps should be taken to safeguard them according to local and national guidelines on child protection. If a professional is aware that a young girl has had the procedure and there are other female children in the family, a referral to social services may be needed following the guidelines. It is important to follow the steps outlined in the Department of Health document on 'What to do if you are worried a child is being abused' (DH, 2003). Women who have had FGM may approach a health professional for advice on reversal in order to restore normal anatomy and some centres in the country provide this service but it is not enough (see list of services given later).

Women who have had FGM in the past may not want to discuss it to a health professional and great harm can be done if a professional shows a reaction on discovering the scars during an examination. Nurses and others working in sexual health should be mindful when examining women from countries where FGM is common practice.

Professionals can ask the women if she has ever had surgery anyway as part of the history and gently seek information about FGM by asking simple questions like 'have you been cut?' Most women will not see FGM as surgery or operation.

FEMININE PAIN

And if I may speak of my wedding night:
I had expected caresses. Sweet kisses. Hugging and love
No. never!
Awaiting me was pain. Suffering and sadness.
I lay in my wedding bed, groaning like a wounded animal, a victim of feminine pain.
At dawn, ridicule awaited me. My mother announced:
Yes, she is a virgin.
When fear gets hold of me.
When anger seizes my body.
When hate becomes my companion, then I get feminine advice,
Because it is only feminine pain. And I am told feminine pain perishes like all feminine things.
The journey continues. Or the struggle continues.
As modern historians say, as the good tie of marriage matures.
As I submit and sorrow subsides, my belly becomes like a balloon
A glimpse of happiness shows, a hope. A new baby. A new life!
But a new life endangers my life.
A baby's birth is death and destruction for me!
It is what my grandmother called the three feminine sorrows.
She said the day of circumcision, the wedding night and the
Birth of a baby are the triple feminine sorrows.
As the birth bursts, I cry for help, when the battered flesh tears.
No mercy. Push! They say. It is only feminine pain.
And now I appeal:
I appeal for love lost, for dreams broken,
For the right to live as a whole human being.
I appeal to all peace loving people to protect, to support and give a hand to innocent little girls who do no harm.
Obedient to their parents and elders, all they know is only smiles.
Initiate them to the world of love, not the world of feminine sorrows.

This poem was written by Dahabo Ali Muse from Somalia and published by Comfort Momoh in her booklet on *Female Genital Mutilation* (2002). Permission was granted by Comfort Momoh MBE FGM/Public Health Specialist to include this poem.

CASE STUDY

A 17 year old woman from Somalia attended a contraceptve clinic and complained about a slight discharge and without considering FGM the doctor proceeded to examine her which caused pain and discomfort. The young women became very upset and demanded to see a different clinician. The doctor who examined her was of Afro-Caribbean origin but born in the United Kingdom and was not familiar with FGM. The young woman expressed her concern that this doctor *ought* to know better. It had to be explained that the doctor was indeed British and educated in a part of the United Kingdom where FGM was not seen in practice. The moral of this tale is that health professionals should be aware of the populations they serve. Victims of FGM and vaginal examinations may be difficult and indeed the woman may be ashamed and unable to explain the procedure in case of shock or ridicule.

CONCLUSION

Having read this chapter the reader should have a better understanding of FGM, understand the law related to FGM and acknowledge the sensitivities of the procedure. Knowledge of national referral services was also provided for the reader.

REFERENCES

International Planned Parenthood Federation (IPPF) (2001), *IPPF Medical Bulletin* statement on female genital mutilation. Vol 35: 1.

Department for Health (2003) What to do if you are worried a child is being abused, London: DH. Available online at www.dh.gov.uk

Department for Education and Skills (DfES) (2004), *Female Genital Mutilation Act 2003: Local Authority Social Services Letter (LASSL 4)*, London: DfES. Available online at www.dfes.gov.uk

Dareer, A. (1983), Epidemiology of female circumcision in the Sudan Tropical Doctor (13): 41–45.

Female Genital Mutilation Act (2003) cited at http://www.hmso.gov.uk/acts

Marjaria, M. (2002), Female Genital Mutilation (FGM). A handbook for health care professionals, available www.shoc@gp-E84025.nhs.uk

Momoh, C. (2000), Female Genital Mutilation – Information for health care professionals, available African Well Woman Clinic Guys hospital London SE1.

Royal College of Nursing (2006), Female Genital Mutilation. Available at www.rcn.org.uk code 003 037 p 8 or by phone to RCN Direct on 0845 772 6100

World Health Organization (1997), Female genital mutilation: a joint WHO/UNICEF/UNFPA statement, Geneva: WHO. Available at www.who.int

World Health Organization (2000), Female genital mutilation. Information fact sheet (241), Geneva: WHO. Available at www.who.int

FURTHER READING

Althus, F. (1997), Female circumcision: rites of passage or violation of rights, *International Family Planning Perspectives*. Vol 23 (3): 130.

Daley, A. (2004), Caring for women who have undergone female genital mutilation, *Nursing Times*. Vol 100 (26): 32.

Department for Education and Skills (DfES) (2004), *Female Genital Mutilation Act 2003: Local Authority Social Services Letter (LASSL 4)*, London: DfES. Available at www.dfes.gov.uk

Lockat, H. (2004), *Female Genital Mutilation*, Oxford: Radcliffe Publishing Group.

Marjaria, M. (2003), Female Genital Mutilation (FGM). Available at malamid@hotmail.com

Momoh, C. (2005), *Female Genital Mutilation*, Oxford: Radcliffe Publishing Group.

World Health Organization (WHO) (2001), A systematic review of the health complications of female genital mutilation including sequelae in childbirth. Geneva: WHO. Available online at www.who.int

World Health Organization (WHO) (2001), *Female Mutilation: The Prevention and the Management of the Health Complications. Policy Guidelines for Nurses and Midwives*. Geneva: WHO. Available at www.who.int

USEFUL ADDRESSES

Services
African Well Woman Clinic
McNair Centre

Guys and St Thomas Hospital
St Thomas Street
London SE1 9RT
Phone: 020 7 955-2381

African Well Woman Clinic
Central Middlesex Hospital
Acton Lane Park Royal
London NW10 7NS
Phone: 020 8965 5733

African Well Woman Clinic
Northwick Park and St Mark's Hospital
Watford Road
Harrow
Middlesex HA1 3UJ
Phone: 020 8869-2870

Birmingham Heartlands Hospital
Princess of Wales Woman's Unit
Labour Ward
Bordesley Green East
Birmingham
Phone: 0121 424 3514

Central Liverpool PCT
FGM Advocacy Worker Rahima Farah
Kuumba Imani Millennium Centre
4 Princess Street
Liverpool L8 1Th
Phone: 051 285 6370

Drop-in Service
Central Health Clinic
1 Mulberry Street
Sheffield 51 2PJ

Organisations
FORWARD (Foundation for Woman's Health Research and
    Development)
Unit 4
765-767-Harrow Road
London NW 10 5NY
www.forwarduk.org.uk

RAINBOW (Research Action and Information Network for the
   Bodily Integrity of Women)
Queens Studios
121 Salisbury Road
London NW 6 6RG

Cervical Screening and HPV Vaccines

11

Kathy French

INTRODUCTION

This chapter will address cervical screening, how the national programme was developed and set up, the procedure involved and possible results. This will be linked to the planned vaccination for the HPV virus which will commence in 2008. The reader will be able to understand the importance of screening and how to access services.

LEARNING OUTCOMES

After reading this chapter the reader should understand the following:

❑ The importance of cervical screening
❑ The possible outcome of a smear test and treatment available
❑ The planned HPV vaccination programme planned for 2008.

BACKGROUND TO THE PROGRAMME

Cervical cancer is the second most common cancer among women worldwide and is the primary cause of cancer-related deaths in women in developing countries. The human papillomavirus (HPV) is a sexually transmitted virus, recognised as the necessary cause of 99% of all cervical cancers. Cervical cancer, unlike many other cancers, is detectable at an earlier stage by well-organised screening programmes. Regular cervical screening and early treatment of precancerous lesions have led to a substantial reduction in cervical cancer in developed countries.

Rates of HPV infection in young women are high following sexual debut and the risk increases with the acquisition of each new sexual partner.

Cervical screening started in the 1960s when a number of local screening programmes were implemented with the help of Medical Officers of Health and enthusiastic cytologists. Other programmes had developed in an *ad hoc* way but there was no clear, effective, well-managed programme within the United Kingdom. Some women at a higher risk of cervical cancer were not screened and those who were screened were not followed up appropriately. Despite the screening programme, there has been a reduction in the death rate from cancer of the cervix in England and Wales between 1950 and 1991, especially in the age group of 55–64 years. Several explanations have been offered for this and one suggestion is that the virus(s) that cause cervical cancer is passed from men to women and this is more prevalent after a world war but this is difficult to confirm. The positive news is that it is worth remembering that cervical mortality in the United Kingdom fell by 40% between 1979 and 1995 according to the Office for National Statistics (Barton-Smith *et al.*, 2003). Approximately, 3000 new cases of cervical cancer are diagnosed each year in England and Wales, resulting in some 1200 deaths (Wakely *et al.*, 2003).

When considering screening for any condition, it is important to consider if the condition is serious enough to warrant the expenditure involved and also if the condition is one where there is an earlier stage of the condition, if diagnosed could then be treated more effectively than at a later stage and cervical screening is one such condition. The changes in the cervix develop over a long period and if changes occur these can be monitored and if necessary treated with excellent results. Wilson and Junger (1960) described 10 principles for screening and these hold true today.

PRINCIPLES OF SCREENING
(1) The condition should pose an important health problem.
(2) The natural history of the disease should be well understood.
(3) There should be a recognisable early stage.
(4) Early treatment should be more beneficial than at a later stage.
(5) There should be a suitable screening test.
(6) The test should be acceptable to the population.

(7) There should be adequate facilities for the diagnosis and treatment of abnormalities detected.

(8) For diseases of insidious onset (such as cervical cancer), screening should be repeated at intervals determined by the natural history of the disease.

(9) The chances of physical/psychological harm must be less than the benefits.

(10) Cost should be balanced against the benefits it provides (Wilson and Junger, 1960) cited in Sutherland (2001).

From the above 10 principles, one can appreciate that screening for cervical cancer fits well into all of them; however, some women still fail to present for screening, some fear that they might get a positive result and others are too embarrassed to have the test. These fears may be based on myths about the procedure or related to religious or cultural beliefs. Nurses and other health care professionals can do a lot to work with these groups of women and their community to explain the benefits and arrange for them to see a female professional if that is an issue for them.

As a result of the national screening programme, death rates due to cervical cancer have fallen markedly in the United Kingdom, from 8.3 per 100,000 women in 1971 to 3.3 per 100,000 in 2005 (Peto *et al.*, 2004).

The National Health Service National Screening Programme (NHSCSP) was set up in 1988 to replace a much uncoordinated approach to screening women for cervical changes. The Department of Health required each health authority in England to introduce a cervical screening programme for all women aged 20–64 years and recommended that the screening should be carried out every 3–5 years. New guidelines later recommend that screening should start at 25 years because the number of positive diagnosis below 20 years is very low.

The first invitation for screening is generated from the GP lists automatically at 25 years and then the woman is part of the recall system every 3 years.

Some Primary Care Trusts continue to screen young women from the age of 20 when they attend a contraception/sexual health clinic if there is a high rate of abnormalities in that population but this is a local decision.

Screening is often confused with a test for 'cancer' and this is not the case, it is not a diagnostic tool but a means of checking for changes in the cervix which may or may not lead to cancer later in life. During 1988, a National Coordinating Network for the NHSCSP was established and this was one of the main successes in the early years of the NHSCSP since it brought together the UK health departments, health authorities, professional bodies and designated mangers to help facilitate the adoption of common standards and working practices throughout the United Kingdom. The publication of the Health of the Nation document in 1992 had an aim to reduce the incidence and mortality rates from cancer of the cervix and a target for the programme to:

- Reduce the incidence of invasive cervical cancer by at least 20% by 2000 from 15 per 1,000,000 population in 1986 to no more than 12 per 1,000,000.

Much progress has been made and especially amongst the older age group (35–64) for whom previous coverage was low but the risk of cervical cancer is relatively high. Cervical screening, although not reaching all women, has been a success. The number of women between 20 and 64 years screened in 1984 was only just over 40% whilst in 1995 over 84% of women had a result within the past 5 years and this high rate has been maintained until fairly recently when numbers have dropped.

For the cervical screening programme to be effective, a National Coordinator was appointed in England to improve the management and quality of the cervical screening programme and similar programmes were put in place in Scotland, Wales and Northern Ireland. The role of the Coordinator was to develop and review national quality standards and national quality initiatives to monitor performance against national standards and to ensure that information is collected to support the evaluation of this national screening programme. This in effect means that at a local level a single individual has overall managerial responsibility for the quality control of the local programme, exercised through contracts and service agreements with relevant providers (NHSCSP, 1996).

Nurses and other health care professionals undertaking cervical screening must be trained in the technique and follow the national screening training programme. It is the responsibility of the smear taker to make every effort to sample the whole of the transformation zone (TZ). The TZ is the part of the cervix where the squamous epithelium and the columnar epithelium of the cervix meet and the cervix must be visualised totally in order to take the smear from the full circumference of the cervix if using the traditional method of screening.

Some of the disadvantages of the conventional smear procedure were poor sampling, poor transfer of the cells, poor spreading of the sample or poor fixation of the cells on the slide. Because of the above-mentioned problems, the National Institute for Health and Clinical Excellence (NICE) recommended that the traditional smear test be replaced by liquid-based cytology (LBC) in 2003. Much anxiety was inflicted upon women who were recalled following a smear because of high numbers of inadequate smears. LBC is being phased into all clinics and Scotland totally relies on LBC. This method of screening differs from sampling the TZ but a special plastic broom-like device is inserted into the endocervical canal where the brush is rotated gently in a clockwise direction and the cellular material is collected. This allows all the material to be retained in the solution and the brush is discarded. The bottle containing the solution is then tightened and sent to the laboratory in a specimen bag according to local protocols.

The procedure should be done according to the manufacturer's instruction. The material is then rinsed in a small plastic vial of preservative solution, either ThinPrep® or SurePath® depending on local decisions. The vial is then transferred to the laboratory. It then comes under an automated process.

LBC has excellent fixation, good cellular detail, clean background, representative cell sample and provide a thin layer of cells over a controlled area. This has resulted in an increased pickup rate of abnormalities, reduced unsatisfactory rate, reduced preparation time and reduced turnaround time.

The results of the smear test are sent to the smear taker, the GP and a letter to the woman informing her of the outcome. The cytologist will report one of the following results:

(A) Normal
(B) Borderline changes
(C) Mild changes, referred to as dyskaryosis or dysplasia

(D) Moderate changes
(E) Severe changes.

Around half (50%) of women with mild changes will revert to a normal over time but will be asked to have their smears repeated sooner than 3 years. This must be explained to women before a smear is taken otherwise some will think they have cancer and will not understand why no treatment is offered.

This is a very stressful time for women, from the time she has decided to have a smear until she gets the results and this can last over a period of many weeks.

Any smear showing moderate or severe changes will be referred for a colposcopy immediately. A colposcopy is performed in an outpatient setting where the cervix is visualised and tissue is taken and analysed by a pathologist and depending on the severity of the changes, either a loop excision is made of the affected area or a wire with an electric current is used to remove the abnormal cells. Cervical screening will take place more frequently following a colposcopy and the woman will not be able to be part of the recall system until she has three consecutive normal smear results.

Should a smear show a positive result to *Trichomonas vaginalis*, the woman should be offered screening for other sexually acquired infections (SAIs) together with any partner. This will need to be handled in a sensitive manner, otherwise great harm could result if a health professional made any allegations about an unfaithful partner. It is important to inform women having a cervical smear what the test is for and indeed what is not included, otherwise some women may think they were screened for many conditions, including cancer of the ovaries, uterus and screened for SAI and HIV. Pelvic bimanual examination is not part of routine cervical screening; women should only be examined if they have symptoms, for example, bleeding, pain or discharge.

It is important to counsel women about possible results and the timescale for getting the results; this can be a time of great concern for some women and telling women that the majority of smears are normal might be helpful. Of the 36 million women screened between 2004 and 2005 in England, the following resulted in:

9.4% were inadequate and needed to be repeated
93% were negative
3.2% showed borderline changes
1.7% showed mild dyskaryosis
0.6% showed moderate dyskaryosis
0.6% showed severe dyskaryosis (Hardy, 2007).

Reflection time

There will be occasions when women refuse or delay having smears and health care professionals can help explore with them about the reasons. It could be that some women have been victims of sexual abuse, had a previous bad experience or from a cultural background where intimate examinations are difficult for them.

VACCINATION AGAINST CERVICAL CANCER

More than 100 virus types of HPV have been described of which at least 35 primary types infect genital epithelium. Some of these viruses are low risk and cause warts whilst others are considered high risk and are involved in the development of cervical cancer. It is thought that 95% of cervical cancers are a result of infection with one or more of the high risk HPV types (Savage and Lowndes, 2006) and about 75% of cancers are caused by HPV types 16 and 18 (Clifford *et al.*, 2003). Several companies

---

CASE SCENARIO

A 26 year old woman using the combined contraceptive pill (COP) attends for a repeat supply of the pill, you notice that she has never had a smear. You suggest she has one soon but she appears to be avoiding that. You look in the medical records and other staff had suggested a smear in the past. Reasons given are 'I have a period now', 'I am in a hurry tonight' or 'I am on my way out with friends'. On further exploration with the woman, she explains that she is frightened to have a smear, a friend told it was very painful and that they might find cancer.

---

have developed a vaccine against HPV and in late 2006, a new vaccine was licensed in the United Kingdom which is considered very effective against HPV types 6, 11, 16 and 18. The Joint Committee on Vaccination and Immunisation, a group of experts in the field, recommended in June 2007 that there is sufficient evidence on the protective effect of HPV vaccines on cervical cancer in the United Kingdom to suggest vaccination of girls between the ages of 12 and 13 as part of the school-based programme in conjunction with a sexual education programme through Personal and Social Education. Clearly, the school nurse teams will play a key role in the delivery of this programme; however, the programme may be school lead but delivered by other teams in areas where the number of school nurses are less. There will of course be some discussion and rhetoric from some sections of the media who will argue that vaccination of young girls will lead to promiscuity but this vaccine should be welcomed as a major advancement for women in the prevention of cervical cancer. This should be seen in the same way as rubella, a vaccination against German measles, and again the reason young girls have this protection is to prevent abnormalities later should they get be in contact with the virus whilst pregnant. One of the safest ways to protect against HPV and other SAIs is by use of condoms and this should be discussed with all sexually active people and be part of any school-based programme on safer sex messages.

Despite having a vaccination available in the future, women will still need to attend for regular screening, as the vaccination programme is only open to teenage girls. The vaccine will not be offered to young men at this point in time and considering that anal carcinoma is linked to the HPV this omission is regretful.

Reflection time
You are told that vaccination of young girls against HPV will lead to promiscuity. How might you address this?

The HPV vaccination should be seen in the same way as other vaccinations, for example, rubella and tuberculosis, and all preventative measures.

CONCLUSION

The chapter addressed the importance of cervical screening, treatment available for abnormal smears and the preventative measures needed to reduce the incidence of cervical cancer. The new HPV vaccination was mentioned and hopefully all practitioners will encourage the use of this new vaccine.

REFERENCES

Barton-Smith, P., Thomas, V. and Ind, T. (2003), Cervical cancer screening in England and Wales: an update, *Reviews in Gynaecological Practice*. Vol 3: 5–10.

Clifford, G.M., Smith, J.S., *et al.* (2003), Human papillomavirus types in invasive cervical cancer worldwide: a meta-analysis, *British Journal of Cancer*. Vol 88 (1): 63.

Hardy, J. (2007), How to take a sample for cervical screening, *Nursing Standard*. Vol 21 (50): 40.

National Health Service Cancer Screening Programmes (NHSCSP) (1996), Quality Assurance Guidelines for the Cervical Screening programme. Available at www.cancerscreening.nhs.uk

Peto, J., Gilham, G., Flethcer, G. and Matthews, F.E. (2004), The cervical cancer epidemic that screening has prevented in the UK, *The Lancet*. Vol 364 (9430): 249.

Savage, E. and Lowndes, C.M. (2006), US study finds that consistent condom use protects against genital human papillomavirus infection. Available at www.eurosurrevielance.org

Sutherland, C. (2001), *Women's Health. A Handbook for Nurses*. Churchill Livingstone, London, p. 24.

Wakely, G., Cunnion, M. and Chambers, R. (2003), *Improving Sexual Health Advice*. Radcliffe Medical Press, Oxon, p. 94.

Wilson, J.M. and Junger, G. (1960), *Principles and Practice of Screening for Disease*. Geneva: World Health Organisation (WHO).

FURTHER READING

Cancer Screening Programme (NHS) (2000), Achievable standards, benchmarks for reporting and criteria for evaluating cervical cytopathology. Available at www.cancerscreening.nhs.uk, Tel 0114271 1060.

Centres for Disease Control and Prevention (2004), Genital HPV infection: CDC fact sheet. Available at www.cdc/gov/std/HPV/STDFact-HPV.htm

Dailard, C. (2006), Achieving universal vaccination against cervical cancer in the United States: The need and the means, *Guttmacher Policy Review*. Vol 9 (4): 1. Available at www.guttmacher.org/pubs/gpr

Department of Health (1999), Bulletin on Cervical Screening Programme. England at www.doh.gov.uk/cervical screening

Homes, K.K., Levine, R. and Weaver, M. (2004), Effectiveness of condoms in preventing sexually transmitted infections, *Bulletin World Health Organisation*. Vol 82 (6): 454 (www.who.int/bulletin/volumes/82/6/454.pdf).

International Planned Parenthood Federation (IPPF) (2007), Medical Bulletin IMAP statement on cervical screening and the role of the human papilloma virus (HPV), Vaccine. Vol 41: 3.

National Institute for Health and Clinical Excellence (2003), Guidance on The Use of Liquid-Based Cytology for Cervical Screening. Technology Appraisal 69. London: NICE.

Quilliam, S. (20060), Cervical cancer and the human papillomavirus vaccine, *The Journal of Family Planning and Reproductive Health Care*. Vol 32 (2): 119.

Royal College of Nursing (2005), Cervical screening RCN guidance for good practice. Available at www.rcn.org.uk or RCN Direct 0845 772 6160 publication code 003 105.

Royal College of Nursing (2006), Human papilloma virus (HPV) and cervical cancer – the facts at www.rcn.otg.uk code 003 083

Sasieni, P., Adams, J. and Cuzick, J. (2003), Benefit of cervical screening at different ages: Evidence from the UK audit of screening histories, *British Journal of Cancer*. Vol 89 (1): 88.

Smith, J.S., Green, J., Berrington de Gonalez, Appleby, P. and Julian, P. (2003), Cervical cancer and use of hormonal contraceptives, *The Lancet*. Vol 361: 1159.

Williams, A. (2006), Does liquid-based cytology really offer any advantage? *The Journal of Family Planning and Reproductive Health Care*. Vol 32 (3): 149.

Winer, R.L., Lee, S.K. *et al.* (2003), Genital human papillomavirus infection: incidence and risk factors in a cohort of human university students, *American Journal of Epidemiology*. Vol 157 (3): 218–226.

USEFUL WEBSITES

www.dh.gov.uk
www.cancerscreening.nhs.uk/cervical/publications/in-04.html
www.colposcopy.org.uk

Training for Nurses and Others in Sexual Health

INTRODUCTION

Student nurses are often forgotten about in terms of sexual health training and many post-registration nurses are often denied the opportunity to gain knowledge and skills in the field. Some manager believing that sexual health has nothing to do with the client/patient being cared for in that speciality.

Sexual health is part of holistic care and should be part of all training for nurses and midwives. Students should demand to have sexual health as part of their training and have the opportunity to visit local sexual health clinics. Nurses who want to gain skills may be able to do so by undertaking contraception/sexual health courses and these are listed at www.guna.org.uk. Sexual health services/clinics can be found at www.bashh.org.uk.

LEARNING OUTCOMES

This brief section will highlight the training needed to work in sexual health.

The Faculty of Sexual and Reproductive Healthcare provides a 2-day course in contraception and many nurses access that module. For nurses wanting to gain skills in genitourinary medicine, they should also check out courses at www.guna.org.uk. The British Association for Sexual Health and AIDS (BASHH) provides a 2-day course throughout the United Kingdom titled the STIF course. This is a sexually transmitted infection foundation course and again many nurses access this module and these are recommended.

Nurses in primary care are often expected to deliver on sexual health without the language, knowledge or skills to help them.

The Royal College of Nursing (RCN) distance learning skills course covered most aspects of sexual health and as from September 2008, this will be available from Greenwich University as an e-learning activity. To date, some 1800 nurses have taken part in this double module programme.

The Royal College of General Practitioners are also drafting an e-learning introduction to sexual health and this should be available early spring 2008.

A2Z of health are planning to launch an e-learning programme for nurses very soon and this will be a basic introduction to sexual health and all these programmes are a welcome addition to existing programmes.

Nurses wanting to train in the fitting of IUDs and sub-dermal implants should follow the RCN guidelines available form RCN Direct at www.rcn.org.uk/sexualhealth.

The Royal College of General Practitioner (RCPG) and others are currently developing an e-learning introduction certificate in sexual health which is planned for 2008.

Those professionals wanting to move into sexual health adviser's roles should check training on www.sha.org.uk.

Non-registered health workers can access excellent training through the fpa and this is available at www.fpa.org.uk.

There are many study days and conferences provided by various organisations and these are often advertised on the GUNA website at www.guna.org.uk

GUNA, BASHH, FSPH, RCN, NANCSH and NIVHNA provide annual conferences and check their websites for dates and topics. List of websites are listed on page 217.

Useful Websites Related to Sexual Health

www.bashh.org.uk	Provides policy and guidelines for SAIs and HIV
www.brook.org.uk	Young peoples services
www.cancerscreening.nhs.uk	Caner screening
www.colposcopy.org.uk	Colposcopy information
www.cdc.gov	Centre for disease control
www.fsrh.org	Guidelines and up-to-date publications on all contraceptive methods
www.fpa.org.uk	Charity for sexual health, advocates for men and women and offers excellent training in sexual health
www.dh.gov.uk	All DH documents on sexual health
www.gmc.org.uk	General Medical Council
www.guna.org.uk	Nursing organisation for sexual health nurses in GUM
www.herpesalliance.org	Herpes international
www.hpa.org.uk	Epidemiology on SAIs and HIV
www.medfash.org.uk	Standards in sexual health and HIV
www.nmc.org.uk	Nursing and Midwifery Council
www.nancsh.org.uk	Nursing organisation for sexual health

www.nmc.org.uk	Standards, codes of practice, medicines management, fit for practice and other useful documents
www.nice.org.uk	Centre for Health and Clinical Excellence
www.nhivna.org.uk	Nursing organisation dealing with HIV
www.rcn.org.uk	Nursing organisation with a sexual health forum
www.rcog.org.uk	Royal College of Obstriticians and Gynaecologists
www.tht.org.uk	Terrence Higgins Trust a Voluntary organisation for HIV/AIDS
www.who.int	World Health Organization

Index